Research Methodology for Allied Health Professionals

Animesh Hazari

Research Methodology for Allied Health Professionals

A comprehensive guide to Thesis & Dissertation

Springer

Animesh Hazari
College of Health Sciences
Gulf Medical University
Ajman, Ajman, United Arab Emirates

ISBN 978-981-99-8924-9 ISBN 978-981-99-8925-6 (eBook)
https://doi.org/10.1007/978-981-99-8925-6

This Springer imprint is published by the registered company Springer Nature Singapore Pte Ltd.
The registered company address is: 152 Beach Road, #21-01/04 Gateway East, Singapore 189721, Singapore

Paper in this product is recyclable.

Foreword

Research methodology plays a pivotal role in the curricula of Allied Health Professionals, serving as the backbone for evidence-based practice and ensuring high-quality healthcare delivery. In the rapidly evolving healthcare field, professionals need to understand the intricacies of research design, data collection, and analysis to make informed decisions. The inclusion of research methodology in Allied Health Professionals' curricula fosters critical thinking and problem-solving skills. It equips students with the ability to evaluate and apply existing research to clinical practice, enabling them to stay updated on the latest advancements and best practices. Moreover, a solid foundation in research methodology empowers Allied Health Professionals to contribute to the growing body of knowledge in their respective fields, addressing gaps in understanding and proposing innovative solutions. By emphasizing research methodology, educational programs ensure that future healthcare practitioners can navigate and contribute to evidence-based literature, enhancing the overall quality and effectiveness of patient care. This integration also promotes a culture of continuous improvement, encouraging Allied Health Professionals to question, explore, and refine their approaches better to meet the diverse needs of patients and communities. Ultimately, research methodology stands as a cornerstone in Allied Health Professionals' education, aligning their skills with the evolving landscape of healthcare and reinforcing the commitment to delivering evidence-based, patient-centered care. With two decades of expertise in Research Methodology, I specialize in clinical and sports biomechanics, gait analysis, and 3D motion capture. As a dedicated professional at Robert Gordon University in the UK, my work revolves around advancements in Allied Health streams through rigorous research. My projects aim to contribute to the academic landscape but also directly impact clinical and sports applications. Through the integration of cutting-edge technology like 3D motion capture, I strive to enhance the precision and depth of biomechanical studies, fostering a culture of innovation and excellence in both research and Allied Health. Based on my academic experience I firmly believe that Dr. Animesh Hazari's book, *Research Methodology for Allied Health Professionals: A Comprehensive Guide to Thesis and Dissertation*, stands as a commendable contribution to the field. Drawing upon his extensive expertise in research methodology, Dr. Hazari provides a valuable resource for Allied Health Professionals navigating the intricacies of thesis and dissertation work. The book is a beacon for students and practitioners alike, offering practical insights and a comprehensive understanding of research methodologies tailored to the unique demands of the Allied Health field. By synthesizing years of experience and expertise, Dr. Hazari elevates the discourse surrounding research methodology in this context. His work not only enriches the academic landscape but also empowers Allied Health Professionals to conduct impactful research, fostering a culture of excellence and innovation in the pursuit of evidence-based practice. The book is a testament to Dr. Hazari's commitment to advancing both the theoretical and practical dimensions of research methodology in Allied Health.

Robert Gordon University Scotland Ioannis Agouris
Aberdeen, UK

Preface

The idea of writing a book on "research methodology" engendered from being a student myself when my supervisor asked me to prepare the research proposal for the master's degree. I was "lost" and searching web on how to conduct research, which made me more confused with given terminologies and different approaches. I did not know how to deal with it, and multiple nights passed by just looking for a start. The supervisor expected just to complete the proposal for the time being and continue working on it, but I believed it was a lot for asking. I read multiple books on research methodology, and I realized that you cannot learn research methodology just as a subject in the curriculum; it demands personal experience. Somehow, I managed to write a proposal and submit, but the task became more difficult in execution as I realized that all I proposed does not seem to be practically applicable in my research project. Thus, the notion of just writing a proposal without understanding the entire process of research methodology is not just stupid but harmful as well, in particular, when we are dealing with human and animal lives. The implications and effects of our research outcome are of high importance. It took me around 2 years to grab the nag of conducting quality research, and I could imply it well during my Ph.D. where I learnt more advanced aspects of research methodology. Ultimately, I gained the requisite experience through conducting various research projects myself and supervising students. When I started teaching the subject, I found those very similary "lost" faces like mine in the class, and then I decided that I will put down my experience of research methodology to help those students in a systematic, stepwise approach to learning research methodology. There are multiple books and literature for research methodology, but they all focus on the theoretical aspect with just defining the terminology without connecting them into practical applications. Students often know the research methods on paper but find it difficult to execute their research projects practically. This book is different in terms of the fact that every chapter has been sequentially put in such a way that if one goes through it, he/she would easily understand the entire process of conducting their research with confidence and accuracy. The book is focused on allied health professionals with citation of multiple examples and scenarios to make them correlate with their own research ideas and modify accordingly. With my great pleasure, I wish that this book would be helpful to all my students and peer researchers to flourish in the research academia with their valuable contribution.

Knowing research is less meaningful than doing!

Ajman, United Arab Emirates Animesh Hazari

Acknowledgments

I would like to put forward my sincere gratitude to all my mentors, supervisors, and research associates for a valuable contribution to my research journey. My special thanks to Prof. Ioannis Agouris (Robert Gordon University, Scotland, UK), Prof. Arun Maiya (Manipal Academy of Higher Education, India), Dr. A.P.S. Bindra (Abhinav Bindra Sports Medicine and Research Institute, India), Prof. Monica Gulati (Lovely Professor University, India), Dr. Praveen Kumar, Prof. Manda Venkatramana, and Prof. Hossam Hamdy (Gulf Medical University, UAE) for their extended support and appreciation in my research career.

I would like to acknowledge Dr. Thumbay Moideen (President, Gulf Medical University, UAE) for giving me an opportunity to continue my contribution as faculty towards academia and research to humankind at Gulf Medical University, UAE. His unmatchable achievements with grace and humbleness have always been inspiring to me, and I look to strive forward every day.

I would like to acknowledge my family, Mr. Krishna Kumar Hazari (father), Mrs. Rita Hazari (mother), Mrs. Rakhi Hazari (wife), and Ms. Anika (daughter), for their immense support at every phase of life. I would have been nothing without them. Sincere thanks to my friends Mr. Pankaj Mishra, Mr. Debasis Goon, Mr. Hafiz Wani, Mr. Ram Shimple, and Mr. Shamim Ahmed who stood beside my abilities and motivated to complete this project with their kind love and companionship.

Finally, I do not find myself complete without the blessing of the Almighty and truly acknowledge their showers of love and blessings. Being most close to my soul, may Lord Shiva always render appreciation for my good deeds!

Animesh Hazari

Contents

Chapter 1
Introduction to Research Methodology

1.1 Overview

The term "research methodology" most often echoes among students, research scholars, and faculty members. Though the application of research methodology is diverse, we shall focus on the content specific to academia and industry. This book would be most helpful to health science students and allow them to learn the process of research in a simple and step-by-step process. In my personal experience, I have found that students are very apprehensive when it comes to learning research methodology as a subject. They often encounter problems in understanding the research methodology as the process starts and throughout the course. At times, they may have completed their research but failed to understand the whole process of how scientifically it was conducted.

1.2 Defining Research Methodology

It is an essential process of any scientific study, which serves as a framework for processing and achieving the predicted outcomes of the study. It is commonly defined as a systematic and organized process of collecting, analyzing, interpreting, and presenting information to answer specific questions or solve problems. It is a vital component of the scientific method and plays a crucial role in advancing knowledge in various fields, such as science, geography, astronomy, humanities, and technology. In this chapter, we will try to give a general overview of the research methodology and its significance.

A. Hazari, *Research Methodology for Allied Health Professionals*,
https://doi.org/10.1007/978-981-99-8925-6_1

1.3 Significance of Research Methodology

The process of research methodology has crucial significance to scientific research with a wide application to academia and industry. The process of sound research methods plays a pivotal role in producing valid and meaningful research outcomes. It establishes the foundation for effective data collection, analysis, and interpretation, ensuring that research findings are reliable. A well-designed research methodology also enhances the reproducibility of research, allowing other researchers to replicate and validate the study's result. The few most common significances have been listed below:

1.3.1 Advancing Knowledge

A well-defined research methodology is a foundation upon which scientific understanding is built and contributes to the expansion of knowledge by discovering new facts, uncovering relationships between two or more variables, and refining existing theories. For example, the current scientific understanding of "big bang theory" is being redefined with the advanced findings from the James Webb Telescope. It may be general information to the public domain; however, it is important to understand that any conclusion made upon this would have, and will undergo rigorous scientific research methods.

1.3.2 Problem-Solving

Research helps identify and address real-world problems and challenges. It provides evidence-based solutions to issues faced by individuals, organizations, and society. For example, if one decides to identify the correct dose of a new drug to treat diabetes effectively, he/she has to conduct research on real patients suffering from the disease and then study the effect of the drug.

1.3.3 Decision-Making

Research findings are required to make an informed choice and decision. For example, a health policy prepared by the government health agencies for "Covid relief and prevention" would require a systematic research process. In addition, the policy of one country would differ from the other due to various factors, which indeed have been further researched. Therefore, if you are a part of such an organization, or have the responsibility to contribute directly or indirectly where a decision has to be made, well-defined research needs to be conducted.

1.3.4 Validating Claims

Research allows for the validation or refutation of claims, ensuring that information is accurate. For example, a pharmaceutical company claims that they have produced a drug to control cancer. The drug would require going through a process of extensive research and testing before this claim could be validated.

1.4 Key Components of Research Methodology

The research methodology encompasses several essential components, each contributing to the overall research process. These components include formulating a hypothesis, research design, sampling techniques, data collection methods, data analysis procedures, and ethical considerations. Understanding these components is vital for researchers to design and execute their studies effectively. In the subsequent chapters, we will learn each component in detail.

1.5 Research Approaches

There could be various approaches to research depending on the nature of the research question and the available resources. It commonly includes quantitative, qualitative, and mixed-method research. Each has its strengths and weaknesses; we will learn about them in the upcoming chapter.

1.6 Research Design

The research design is a fundamental aspect of research methodology, outlining the overall strategy and structure of the study. It includes decisions regarding the research type (e.g., descriptive, experimental), the selection of variables, and the determination of the study's scope and timeframe. We must carefully consider the design to ensure that the study aligns with their research objectives. These designs will be explained in detail with suitable examples in the upcoming chapters.

1.7 Types of Research

The research types are classified as follows:

1.7.1 Basic Research

This type of research is conducted to expand fundamental knowledge and understanding in a particular field without any immediate or specific application. Basic research contributes to the development of theories and concepts.

1.7.2 Applied Research

Applied research aims to address specific practical problems and provides solutions to real-world issues. It often builds upon the findings of basic research and seeks to apply them in practical contexts.

1.7.3 Quantitative Research

In quantitative research, data is collected in numerical form and analyzed using statistical methods. Researchers use surveys, experiments, or structured observations to gather data.

1.7.4 Qualitative Research

Qualitative research focuses on understanding and interpreting non-numerical data, such as interviews, focus groups, case studies, and observations. It aims to explore complex phenomena and gain an in-depth understanding of social behavior and experiences.

1.8 Research Process

The process of research follows a systematic and stepwise execution of tasks as listed below. Each process will be described in detail in the upcoming chapters.

1.8.1 Formulating Research Questions

The first step in any research project is to define clear and specific research questions or objectives. These questions guide the entire research process.

1.8.2 Literature Review

Researchers conduct a comprehensive review of existing literature and studies related to their topic. This step helps them understand what has already been explored, identify gaps in knowledge, and refine their research questions.

1.8.3 Research Design

Researchers choose an appropriate research design, which includes selecting the methods and procedures to collect and analyze data. The design should align with the research questions and objectives.

1.8.4 Data Collection

This step involves gathering data using methods such as surveys, experiments, interviews, or observations. Researchers should ensure data quality and reliability.

1.8.5 Data Analysis

Once the data is collected, it is analyzed using appropriate statistical or qualitative techniques, depending on the research design.

1.8.6 Drawing Conclusions

Researchers interpret the results of the data analysis and draw conclusions based on the evidence gathered during the study.

1.8.7 Reporting and Dissemination

The final step involves communicating the research findings through academic papers, reports, conferences, or other appropriate channels.

1.9 Summary

Research is a powerful tool for acquiring knowledge, solving problems, and making informed decisions. Understanding the significance of research, and steps involved can help researchers conduct meaningful studies that contribute to the advancement of knowledge thereby benefiting society. This chapter introduces research methodology, highlighting its importance and key components. By understanding research methodology, researchers can design and conduct studies that yield reliable and valid results. The subsequent chapters of this book will deliver deeper insights into each component of research methodology, equipping researchers with the knowledge and skills necessary for conducting high-quality research.

Chapter 2
Application of Research Methodology in Allied Health Profession: Thesis and Dissertation

2.1 Thesis and Dissertation

The terms "thesis" and "dissertation" are often used interchangeably, but in some contexts, they can have different meanings. The main difference between the two lies in their usage and the level of study at which they are accomplished.

2.1.1 Thesis

A thesis is usually associated with a master's degree program. It is a formal academic paper that presents original research conducted by the student under the guidance of a faculty advisor. In a thesis, the student explores a specific research question, problem, or topic and provides a detailed analysis of the subject matter. The thesis should demonstrate the student's ability to conduct independent research, analyze data, and draw meaningful conclusions. They are generally shorter than dissertations in terms of presentation as well as a timeline for conduction.

2.1.2 Dissertation

A dissertation is typically associated with a doctoral (Ph.D.) degree program. It is a comprehensive and in-depth piece of original research that contributes new knowledge to the field. Dissertations are much more extensive and rigorous. They require the student to conduct extensive research, demonstrate expertise in the subject area, and contribute novel insights or theories to the academic community.

A. Hazari, *Research Methodology for Allied Health Professionals*,
https://doi.org/10.1007/978-981-99-8925-6_2

While these differences are generally observed, the terminology can vary depending on the country, educational institution, or academic discipline. For example, in some countries, the term "thesis" is used for both master's and doctoral level research.

2.2 Research Methodology in Health Organizations

Research in health organizations has a major role to play wherein best practices are implemented based on scientific evidence. A health organization can be well recognized by the type and quality of research output, and indeed recognition and accreditation are achieved. A health organization could be a center of research for external funding, and multiple trials could be conducted. To be an established research center for health, the organization needs to be well equipped and have sufficient resources to conduct the research with the most accuracy. The World Health Organization has its distinguished research centers for health to conduct research under various domains and objectives. Therefore, the role of research in health organizations is of prime importance for the welfare and betterment of health services.

2.3 Research Methodology in Academia

The role of research in academia gains high significance for students, research scholars, and faculty members. Research and development is an important department for any academic organization, which helps to enhance the research output in terms of paper publication, copyrights, grants, funding opportunities, etc. In addition, research is an essential component of institutional ranking and accreditation. The research methodology as a part of the curriculum in the academic setup helps and allows students to understand the process of conducting research in detail. The assessment is extensive through the thesis and dissertation. The research methodology is an important course of the curriculum for the award of a degree. Therefore, we must learn all the components of research methodology well enough to complete our research thesis or dissertation.

2.4 Research Methodology in Allied Health Profession: Thesis and Dissertation

Research methodology plays a crucial role in the field of allied health professions when it comes to conducting thesis and dissertation studies. Allied health professions encompass a broad range of healthcare disciplines, including physical therapy, occupational therapy, nursing, radiology, speech-language pathology, and more. Here are some key aspects of the research methodology applied in allied health profession thesis and dissertation studies.

2.4.1 Research Methodology in Physical Therapy

A physical therapist can apply the concepts of research methodology to understand the effectiveness of a particular exercise regimen or interventional program. For example, we currently know that cardiovascular endurance can be trained through aerobic exercises. How could that be concluded? To establish this fact, research needs to be done with various types of exercise regimens, given to a specific population, and study the effects of each exercise type. Based on the statistical and clinical significance, it could be suggested that among all types of exercises, the aerobic exercise regime has the maximum effects on training cardiovascular endurance. Various such findings could be done in the field of physical therapy.

2.4.2 Research Methodology in Medical Lab Sciences

A medical laboratory science student could determine the most effective biochemistry test for the detection of certain disorders using the process of research methodology. For example, we currently know that HbA1c is the most reliable parameter to detect hyperglycemia compared to fasting blood sugar (FBS) and postprandial blood sugar (PPBS). How could this be achieved? Researches would have been conducted to compare and correlate the HbA1c, FBS, and PPBS with the hyperglycemic status of subjects to conclude the highest statistical and clinical relevance for HbA1c.

2.4.3 Research Methodology in Medical Imaging Sciences

A medical imaging science student could determine the most effective radiological test for the detection of certain disorders using the process of research methodology. For example, we currently know that soft tissue disorders could be best studied through medical resonance imaging (MRI) techniques compared to an X-ray. This could also be concluded through research conducted to compare the findings of a soft tissue injury on the MRI and X-ray, respectively.

Similarly, all other allied health professionals could apply the research methodology in their specific areas of expertise. All allied health professionals follow a standard procedure of research methodology. It is important to note that the specific application of research methodology in allied health thesis and dissertation studies may vary depending on the discipline, research focus, and individual research project. Researchers should consult relevant research textbooks, methodological literature, and their academic advisors for guidance specific to their field.

Chapter 3
Components of Research Methodology

3.1 Background

This chapter gives an overall understanding of components used in any research sequentially. These components would be followed and used for conducting as well as writing the research projects. In my personal experience, it would lead the readers to conduct their research projects with accuracy and scientific rigor. Here, we will try to list the components and briefly discuss them. Detailed information will be given in the chapters ahead. These components of research methodology can vary depending on the field of study and the research design, but here are the key components commonly found in most research methodologies:

3.1.1 Research Philosophy

Also known as the "research paradigm" which guides the researcher's understanding of knowledge and reality. It refers to the set of beliefs, assumptions, and principles that guide the way researchers approach their investigations, frame their questions, interpret their findings, and establish the validity of their work. It serves as a foundational framework that shapes the entire research process, from the formulation of hypotheses to the selection of methodologies and the interpretation of results. The research paradigm helps define the overall research approach and influences how researchers would gather and analyze data. Some of the most prominent research paradigms include the following:

A. Hazari, *Research Methodology for Allied Health Professionals*,
https://doi.org/10.1007/978-981-99-8925-6_3

3.1.1.1 Positivism

The researcher's intent to uncover objective truths by using quantitative methods to measure and analyze a phenomenon. They often emphasize control, objectivity, and replicability in their research. For example, a physical therapist's intent is to assess how effective is the application of laser therapy in musculoskeletal conditions like arthritis. The research paradigm has a positive perception that laser would be effective, and accordingly, research approach, design, and objectives would be set to get the desired results.

3.1.1.2 Interpretivism

It is also known as constructivism or phenomenology and emphasizes the importance of understanding how individuals perceive and interpret the world (subjective). Researchers following this paradigm often use qualitative methods to explore the experiences of participants. They focus on context, cultural influences, and personal interpretations. For example, an allied health student wants to understand the perception and believes of people towards Covid-19 vaccination.

3.1.1.3 Critical Theory

In this paradigm, we analyze and critique existing social systems, seeking to bring about social change and empowerment. Critical research often employs qualitative methods. For example, a researcher wants to check the quality of health services to its employees by a government organization.

3.1.1.4 Pragmatism

Pragmatism combines elements of positivism and interpretivism, focusing on practical solutions to real-world problems. Researchers in this paradigm prioritize the usefulness of research findings and may employ a mix of quantitative and qualitative methods to address complex issues.

3.1.1.5 Constructivism

It emphasizes the idea that knowledge is constructed by individuals based on their experiences and interactions. This paradigm is often associated with qualitative research methods. For example, a researcher wants to understand the behavior of gravity on the planet Mars. The researcher would seek information from previous knowledge and thus construct ways to conclude.

Note: It is important to note that researchers are not strictly bound to a single paradigm, and there is often overlap and flexibility in how paradigms are applied. The choice of research paradigm depends on the research question, the nature of the phenomenon being studied, and the researcher's own beliefs and values.

3.1.2 Research Design

The research design outlines the plan for the study, including the research strategy, data collection methods, and data analysis techniques. Broadly, research designs are categorized into experimental and observational studies, which are well explained in Chap. 5.

3.1.3 Research Approach

This pertains to the overall strategy used to address the research problem. It could be quantitative, qualitative, or mixed methods. Quantitative research involves collecting and analyzing numerical data, while qualitative research focuses on nonnumerical data like text, images, or observations. The mixed method implies to combination of quantitative and qualitative approach.

3.1.4 Review of Literature

This involves finding the existing knowledge in the previous study to draw a hypothesis for the desired study. It helps to avoid duplication of research work and enables the researchers to add to the existing knowledge. The entire process of conducting a review of literature is focused on identifying the ***"research gap."*** The review of literature is conducted in a systematic order using literature search engines and databases. "How to conduct a literature search" has been discussed separately in the upcoming chapters. Let us understand the research gap analysis here.

Research gap analysis is a critical step in the research process that involves identifying areas where current knowledge or understanding is lacking, thereby providing opportunities for new research to contribute valuable insights. There are several types of research gap analysis that researchers can conduct:

3.1.4.1 Conceptual Gap Analysis

This type of gap analysis focuses on identifying gaps in definitions, and concepts within a particular field. Researchers examine existing literature to determine if there are inconsistencies, ambiguities, or unresolved issues in the conceptual framework of a topic. For example, a researcher wants to check the efficacy of Mulligan mobilization in rheumatoid arthritis.

3.1.4.2 Empirical Gap Analysis

Empirical gap analysis involves identifying gaps in empirical evidence or data related to a specific research question. Researchers assess whether there is a lack of studies, insufficient sample sizes, or a lack of evidence used to investigate a particular phenomenon.

3.1.4.3 Methodological Gap Analysis

Methodological gaps refer to areas where existing research methods are inadequate or where innovative approaches could yield better results. Researchers assess whether there are limitations in the methods, tools, or techniques commonly employed in a specific field.

3.1.4.4 Theoretical Gap Analysis

This type of gap analysis involves identifying gaps in existing theoretical frameworks and models. Researchers examine whether there are unexplored aspects, contradictions, or opportunities to refine and expand existing theories.

3.1.4.5 Geographical or Cultural Gap Analysis

Geographical or cultural gap analysis focuses on identifying research gaps that pertain to specific geographic regions or cultural contexts. Researchers assess whether certain populations or regions are underrepresented in the literature, limiting the generalizability of findings.

3.1.4.6 Interdisciplinary Gap Analysis

Interdisciplinary gap analysis involves identifying areas where insights from multiple disciplines could contribute to a more comprehensive understanding of a topic. Researchers assess whether collaboration between different fields could lead to new perspectives and solutions.

3.1.4.7 Policy and Practical Gap Analysis

In this type of gap analysis, researchers identify gaps between research findings and their application in policy or practice. This involves assessing whether research outcomes are effectively influencing decision-making and real-world applications.

3.1.4.8 Temporal Gap Analysis

Temporal gap analysis involves identifying gaps in the research timeline, where there may be historical gaps in understanding or where trends and changes over time have not been adequately explored.

3.1.4.9 Technology Gap Analysis

This type of gap analysis focuses on identifying areas where advancements in technology could lead to new research opportunities or solutions. Researchers assess whether emerging technologies could enhance data collection, analysis, or presentation of findings.

3.1.4.10 Ethical and Social Gap Analysis

Ethical and social gap analysis involves identifying research gaps that address ethical concerns, social implications, or the potential impact of research on various stakeholders. Researchers assess whether ethical considerations and social consequences are adequately addressed in the literature.

Note: When conducting a research gap analysis, researchers typically review existing literature, identify areas of uncertainty or unexplored terrain, and then formulate research questions or hypotheses that aim to address these gaps. This process helps ensure that the new research contributes meaningfully to the advancement of knowledge and addresses relevant challenges within the field.

3.1.5 Sampling Strategy

This involves determining how the research sample (a subset of the population) will be selected. The goal is to ensure that the sample is representative of the larger population to generalize from the findings. The types of sampling and methods have been discussed in detail in Chap. 6.

3.1.6 Data Collection Tools/Instrumentation

These are the techniques used to gather relevant data for the study. They could be in the form of questionnaires, scales, advanced equipment, etc. often referred to as **"research outcome measures."** In research, it includes details about their development, validation, and reliability.

The ***validity*** of an instrument is determined by its accuracy to provide the desired variable. For example, the goniometer is a valid tool to measure joint range of motion but not a valid tool for measuring muscle strength. Similarly, spirometry is a valid tool to measure the oxygen saturation in an individual but not a valid tool to determine the hemoglobin level.

The ***reliability*** of an instrument refers to its ability to produce the same result multiple times of application. For example, the reliability of the goniometer is less compared to the 3D motion analysis systems; however, both are valid tools for joint range of motion analysis. The reliability of an instrument is also influenced by differences in the technique between and among the researchers. For example, one researcher used goniometry to find the shoulder joint range of motion and recorded 170 degrees of shoulder flexion in a frozen shoulder patient. The same researcher does it next time and records 168 degrees of shoulder flexion; this would be known as ***intra-rater reliability.*** The difference between the two different researchers would be known as ***inter-rater reliability***. The outcome measures/instruments are used to collect outcome variables using various data collection methods such as surveys, interviews, observations, experiments, content analysis, and archival research. The data variables should be documented in a data sheet for each participant.

3.1.7 Data Analysis Methods

This involves processing and interpreting the collected data to draw meaningful conclusions. Quantitative data might be analyzed using statistical techniques (SPSS, Excel, R software, etc.), while qualitative data may involve thematic analysis, content analysis, or discourse analysis.

3.1.8 Ethical Considerations

Research ethics involve ensuring that the rights and well-being of research participants are protected. This includes obtaining informed consent, maintaining privacy and confidentiality, and minimizing any potential harm through providing a well-documented participant information sheet.

3.1.9 Data Interpretation

This involves a meaningful representation of collected data, intending to conclude, and relates the findings to the research questions or hypotheses.

3.1.10 Research Limitations

It should be well understood that no research is complete in its form, and therefore it is important to acknowledge the limitations of the study, such as constraints in sample size, scope, or methodology, which might affect the generalizability of the findings.

3.1.11 Results

The results section presents the analyzed data, often using tables, graphs, or statistical summaries.

3.1.12 Conclusion

The conclusion section summarizes the key findings, discusses their implications, and suggests areas for future research.

3.1.13 References and Citations

Citing the sources of information used in the study is crucial for giving credit to previous research and maintaining academic integrity. Chapter 12 discusses the use of references in detail.

3.1.14 Summary

The research components work together to form a comprehensive research methodology that guides the entire research process, from identifying the research problem to communicating the results. The specific components have been emphasized in the upcoming chapters.

Chapter 4
Formulating Research Hypothesis and Objective

4.1 Background

Formulating a research hypothesis and objectives is the first and foremost step in any research process as they provide a clear direction and purpose for your study. In this chapter, we shall learn about formulating an ideal research hypothesis and objectives. Formulation and development of the hypothesis and objectives take place under the following key steps:

4.1.1 Understanding the Research Area

It is often difficult for any researcher or student to get a start with the research project. The best approach is to choose the area of interest that fascinates you or you think would be willing to work with your heart (remember not to be overambitious). Now the area of research interest is not the same as interest in the program or course. It is a very specified area under which a researcher would like to contribute. You could start with a broader area and then taper it to be more specific and focused. For example, a physical therapist has an interest in the musculoskeletal subject, under the course he/she is willing to research the musculoskeletal aspects of shoulder joints. He/she believes that traumatic injury to the ligaments of the shoulder joint is less explored as per his/her current knowledge of the subject. Now he/she starts working on the research gap in the literature, and then a hypothesis is formulated.

A. Hazari, *Research Methodology for Allied Health Professionals*,
https://doi.org/10.1007/978-981-99-8925-6_4

4.1.2 Identification of the Problem

Identification of the research problem is a linked pathway between the research hypothesis, literature gap, and research objective. Identifying a research problem is similar to identifying any general or social problem, but defining the research problem is more scientific and should be focused on something that has not been answered yet by the existing research or still a significant contribution could be made to it. For example, any stated topic related to Covid-19 could be a potential research problem since the subject has been limitedly explored to date, whereas finding a new research problem in tuberculosis would be quite difficult since it has been well explored through various research in the past two decades and there would be less scope to find a research gap.

4.1.3 Developing a Research Question

Developing a research question could also be referred to as a ***"research statement"*** and refers to a specific, focused question that necessitates conduction of research to answer it. For example: "Does Covid-19 have a higher infection rate among diabetics?" It is a research question that needs to be answered by conducting a research survey. Here, area of research interest is "Covid-19" and the identification of the problem would be "infection caused by Covid-19".

4.1.4 Formulating a Hypothesis

A sound hypothesis is formed based on the above three components. A hypothesis is a guess about the relationship between variables. It predicts an outcome that you can test through research. There are two types of hypotheses:

4.1.4.1 Null Hypothesis (H0)

States that there is no significant relationship between the variables.

4.1.4.2 Alternate Hypothesis (H1)

States the specific relationship we expect to find. It is the opposite of the null hypothesis.

Example 4.1
A Physical Therapy student has an interest studying the difference in Quadriceps and Hamstring muscle strength among elite footballers. Let us formulate the research hypothesis for this proposed research.

Area of interest: musculoskeletal condition in elite footballers

Identification of problem: muscular strength difference

Research question: whether a strength difference exists between the flexors and extensors

Null hypothesis: There is no statistically significant difference in muscle strength between quadriceps and hamstrings among elite footballers.

Alternate hypothesis: There is a statistically significant difference in muscle strength between quadriceps and hamstrings among elite footballers.

Example 4.2
A Medical lab master's student has an interest in studying the effects of Salmonella infection on liver enzymes. Let us formulate the research hypothesis for this proposed research.

Area of interest: liver enzymes/salmonella

Identification of problem: infection caused by salmonella

Research question: whether the infection caused by salmonella could affect the levels of liver enzymes

Null hypothesis: There is no statistically significant change in the levels of liver enzymes with salmonella infection.

Alternate hypothesis: There is a statistically significant change in the levels of liver enzymes with salmonella infection.

4.1.5 Designing Research Objectives

Research objectives are specific steps to test your hypothesis and answer your research question. Research objectives are often classified into:

Primary objective: The main objective of the research is broken into specific, smaller, and manageable tasks.

Secondary objective: This could be an additional objective not stated otherwise.

4.1.5.1 Criteria for Designing Good Research Objectives: SMART Criteria

An objective should be

- **S**pecific
- **M**easurable
- **A**chievable
- **R**elevant
- **T**ime-bound (SMART)

Example 4.3
A physical therapy student is researching the effects of a new exercise program on obesity among females.

The research question could be: "Does using a new exercise program improve weight management strategies in obese females?"

The hypothesis could be: "Obese females who use the new exercise program could manage their weight more efficiently than those who do not use the program."

Our objectives could be:

Primary objective: To determine the effects of the exercise program on weight management in obese females

Secondary objective: To correlate physical activity with weight management in obese females.

Example 4.4
A medical imaging student is researching the effects of a new technique on the application of CT scans among neurological patients.

The research question could be: "Does using a new technique improve the application of CT scans among neurological patients?"

The hypothesis could be: "New CT imaging techniques could be more beneficial in identifying the course of neurological disorder compared to older techniques."

Task: Design a suitable objective following the SMART criteria.

Note: Both hypotheses and objectives should reflect the scope of your research and guide your entire study. They will help you stay focused and ensure that your research is structured and meaningful.

4.1.6 Summary

Formulating a research hypothesis and objective is an essential and crucial step to start any research project. The objective must follow the SMART criteria to be defined well. Research hypotheses allow a framework on which the entire research methodology could be prepared.

Chapter 5
Research Designs

5.1 Background

In this chapter, we shall learn about various types of research designs. A researcher needs to choose the correct research design based on the plan and requirements of the study. The "research design" refers to the plan or structure that guides the process of conducting a research study. In simple words, it outlines the methods, procedures, and strategies that researchers will use to address their research questions or hypotheses. A well-designed research study should have a clear and logical research design that would enhance the accuracy of data collection, data analysis, and interpretation of results.

5.2 Components of Research Design

All research design has integrated components that form the complete research study.

A research design typically includes the following components:

5.2.1 Research Questions or Hypotheses

Articulated questions or statements that the study aims to address the problem. Examples are given in the previous chapter.

A. Hazari, *Research Methodology for Allied Health Professionals*, https://doi.org/10.1007/978-981-99-8925-6_5

5.2.2 *Research Approach*

Research approaches provide a framework for how researchers gather, analyze, and interpret data in line with the selected research design. The research approaches can be tailored to fit the needs of various allied health professions and their specific research questions. The choice of approach depends on the nature of the research question, available resources, and desired depth of understanding.

The commonly used research approaches have been discussed here.

5.2.2.1 Quantitative Research Approach

Quantitative research involves collecting numerical data and analyzing it using statistical methods to quantify relationships and patterns. In simple words, this approach is taken when the findings of the study need to be presented in numbers, percentages, ratios, etc. This approach is often used to answer research questions that involve measuring variables and examining cause-and-effect relationships.

Example 5.1
A physical therapist wants to determine the prevalence rate of work-related musculoskeletal disorders among the teachers. He would need to put his results into prevalence rate as a percentage, and thus a quantitative approach would be taken.

Example 5.2
A medical laboratory health professional aims to determine the bacterial count in a specimen from tuberculosis patients. He must use the quantitative approach to achieve the number.

Example 5.3
A health professional wants to study the levels of biomarkers used to detect and confirm the diagnosis for a particular disease; he should use the quantitative approach.

5.2.2.2 Qualitative Research Approach

Qualitative research focuses on understanding the underlying meaning and context of phenomena through methods like interviews, observations, and content analysis. It aims to capture participants' perspectives and experiences. When data cannot be represented through numbers, quantitative approaches are taken.

Example 5.4
A physical therapist aims to explore how patients perceive the quality of their treatment for a particular disorder. He will collect qualitative information through an interview or questionnaire from all patients as perseverance cannot be quantified. Qualitative approaches are not used otherwise when quantitative cannot be employed

and are absolute. The reason is that qualitative information lacks accuracy for research purposes and is difficult to provide a distinct conclusion with consistency.

However, ordinal scales or Likert scales could be used to code the data into numbers and present them for easy understanding.

5.2.2.3 Mixed-Methods Approach

This approach involves combining both quantitative and qualitative research methods to provide a comprehensive understanding of a research question. Researchers collect and analyze both numerical and textual data to gain deeper insights.

Example 5.5
A health professional aims to identify and collect quantitative data on the prevalence of Covid-19 among healthcare workers in an outpatient department and qualitative data through conducting interviews to explore the underlying causes and coping strategies.

5.2.3 Variables

Identification of the independent and dependent variables, as well as any potential confounding variables are essential components of research design. Confounding variables refer to the associated factors and variables that would interact with the primary variables and affect the results of the study. For example, you are conducting a study to determine the mental status of a stroke survivor following a traumatic head injury. If the patient is under strong sedative medication, then his mental orientation could be affected and not recorded with accuracy. Therefore, the drug/medication is a confounding variable here and should be taken into consideration. However, there could be instances where the confounding variables cannot be controlled and should be put under the limitations of the study. For example, a batch of physiotherapy students have been given a research project for completion. The study aims to identify the correlation between the duration of work and task output. In this case, there can be multiple confounders that may not be controlled such as help from others to complete the task, individual interest in the subject area, mental abilities, current health status, environmental differences, and socioeconomic status.

5.2.4 Sampling Strategy

Determines how participants or subjects will be selected for the study. This also involves deciding on the sample size and the criteria for inclusion. The strategy for sampling would differ from one research design to another research design. Different methods of sampling have been described with examples in Chap. 6.

5.2.5 Data Collection Methods

Choosing the methods and tools for gathering data. This could involve surveys, interviews, observations, experiments, etc., which has been detailed in Chap. 9.

5.2.6 Data Analysis Techniques

Identifying the statistical or analytical methods that will be used to analyze the collected data. The data analysis using statistical methods has been discussed in Chap. 10.

5.3 Types of Research Designs

The type and choice of research design depend on the research objectives, nature of the research questions, available resources, and ethical considerations. Researchers often need to strike a balance between the rigor of the design and the practicality of its implementation. The research designs are applied to both quantitative and qualitative approaches and are often used in the allied health streams as follows:

5.3.1 Experimental Research Design

This involves manipulation of variables to test the cause-and-effect relationship. For example, a physical therapist aims to determine the effects of resistance exercise training on the blood sugar levels in diabetic patients, or a medical laboratory professional aims to identify the efficacy of a given vaccine on a particular infection. In both instances, the researcher will need to conduct an experiment and manipulate the independent variable to study the effect on the dependent variable. For the physical therapist, the independent variable is resistance exercise, which can be manipulated in frequency, time, intensity, etc., whereas the laboratory professional will try to manipulate the dose and achieve the optimal level to control the infection efficiently. The experimental designs can be further categorized into randomized controlled trials (RCTs) and pre-post designs (non-randomized controlled trials) (Fig. 5.1).

5.3.1.1 Randomized Controlled Trial (RCT)

As the name suggests, it necessarily contains an interventional group and a controlled group. In this type of experimental study design, participants are randomly recruited to an intervention or a control group, and the effects of the intervention are measured.

Example 5.6
A physical therapist wants to study the efficacy of Mulligan exercises over low back pain. The therapist needs to adopt a quantitative approach and experimental research design with RCT. The therapist would select his eligible participants using an appropriate sampling method and then do the process of randomization to select who would receive Mulligan exercise as intervention and who would not be given Mulligan to be considered controlled.

Notes:

1. There is a difference between random sampling and randomized controlled trials, which is most often misunderstood by the researchers. Random sampling means the allocation of participants randomly, whereas RCT refers to the allocation of intervention randomly. If there are only two groups of participants, then

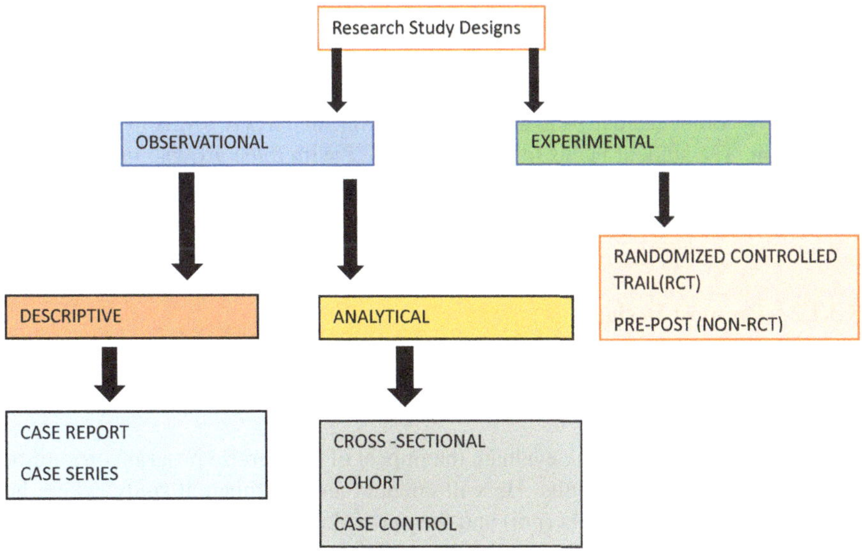

Fig. 5.1 Different types of research study designs

random sampling can correctly be taken as a randomized controlled trial design. For instance, in the above example, there are two groups, "intervention" and "control." If we randomly sample to select the intervention group for the Mulligan exercise, the other group eventually would be controlled, and our random sampling would be enough. However, if we have three groups, random sampling will not suffice. In the above example, consider that the therapist wants to study and compare the Mulligan exercises to the McKenzie exercise for low back pain. The researcher would require three groups here: two interventions (Mulligan and McKenzie) and one control. In this case, the therapist needs to select three different groups from a cohort of back pain patients. He would first do the random sampling and divide the patients into groups A, B, and C within the inclusion criteria. Now he further needs to decide who will be given the Mulligan exercise, who will undertake McKenzie, and who will be kept as the control group with no exercise. For this, he would again do the randomization and allocate the participants to justify the research design as RCT.

2. A control group is a must for RCT as they form the basis for comparison and detect actual change for the given intervention. For example, one may argue that to compare the efficacy of Mulligan to McKenzie, we could directly compare the change in back pain score between the two intervention groups. However, the correct interpretation would be how much change the individual intervention has brought from the baseline, which is only represented by the control group, and since no intervention was given to them, confounding variables would have been controlled.
3. Ethical considerations arise for RCT most often and should be considered. For example, participants in the control group are devoid of intervention, which may not be correct as per the health service commitments. Thus, care should be taken while conducting RCT designs.

Example 5.7
A medical lab student is conducting research and aims to determine the efficacy of 500 mg Glycomet against 1000 mg Glycomet over the HbA1c levels in the diabetic population. The student needs to conduct an RCT with three groups. In one group, he/she would assign Glycomet 500 mg, another group 1000 mg, and the third as the control group.

5.3.1.2 Pre-post Design

Measures are taken before and after an intervention, without a control group.

Example 5.8
A physical therapist wants to evaluate the impact of an exercise program on cardiovascular fitness in older adults. He will conduct an experimental study, where he would first take baseline data (pre) and then provide exercise to the assigned group without randomization followed by collection of data at the end of training (post).

5.3.1.3 Quasi-Experimental Design

It is also known as the "nonequivalent control group design" where participants are assigned to intervention and control groups, but randomization is not possible. For instance, researchers want to assess the effectiveness of a new Covid-19 medication by comparing a group of patients receiving the medication with a similar group receiving standard care. In simple words, true control groups cannot be selected as standard intervention needs to be given due to health concerns.

Example 5.9
A medical laboratory professional wants to detect the efficacy of Pfizer vaccination over the platelet counts in an infected Covid-19 patient. He/she will choose his/her study design as quasi-experimental since one group will be vaccinated to check the effect, but another group also needs health services for active infection. The effectiveness of the intervention (vaccine) would be concluded against the standard care. Since other groups also received some sort of intervention in terms of standard care, the actual difference may be masked to determine the true efficacy of vaccination.

5.3.2 Observational Research Design

This is also known as the "cross-sectional study design" where data is collected at a single point in time, providing characteristics, averages, trends, etc. of a population in a particular geographical area without manipulating the independent variables. Observational studies are further classified into "descriptive" and "analytic" (Fig. 5.1).

Example 5.10 A physical therapist aims to analyze the prevalence of knee osteoarthritis among adult females in the United Arab Emirates. He/she would conduct a cross-sectional study investigating the prevalence rate.

Example 5.11 A medical lab professional wants to know what proportion of people in the United Arab Emirates have blood group A. He/she needs to conduct a survey which is a type of cross-sectional study. As a simple product, one-time blood group testing is required without any intervention, and proportion can be analyzed using a quantitative approach.

5.3.2.1 Cohort Study

Participants are followed over a specific period to examine the development of outcomes or exposures in a homogenous group.

Example 5.12
A physical therapist wants to study the effects of smoking on lung function in a group of healthcare workers. Here, healthcare workers are a cohort of smokers forming a homogenous group (similar characteristics such as smoking).

5.3.2.2 Case-Control Study

Individuals with a specific condition (cases) are compared to those without the condition (controls) to identify factors associated with the condition.

Example 5.13
A medical laboratory professional wants to study the anabolic and catabolic rate of WBC destruction in a typhoid patient compared to a non-typhoid healthy patient.

These are examples of research designs commonly used by allied health professionals. Many other research designs and subcategorization have been proposed in the literature; however, broadly, they fall into either experimental or observational. The choice of design depends on the research question, available resources, ethical considerations, and feasibility.

Chapter 6
Sampling Types and Methods

6.1 Background

Sampling is the process of selecting an ideal sample that would represent the entire population of your desired study. It usually consists of a subset of individuals, items, or data points from a larger population to make inferences or draw conclusions about the entire population. Sampling in research methodology is an important step for participant recruitment once the research hypothesis, objective, and research design have been selected for the given study. The selection of the correct sampling type and method would ensure the accuracy of research data and its results. Sampling is performed before the process of data collection. It should be well understood by the researcher that sampling is different from the sample recruitment process, which often overlaps. Sampling is a prerequisite for the sample recruitment process in research. Sample recruitment is done from the pool of selected samples based on the inclusion and exclusion criteria: for instance, if a researcher wants to conduct a survey on complications of Covid-19 infection among the diabetic population within the age group of 30–40 years. Since this study involves humans, sampling process would initially involve selecting individuals with diabetes mellitus infected with Covid-19. However, the final participants' recruitment would consist of an age group of 30–40 years, which is an inclusion criterion. There are various types of sampling methods that researchers can use to ensure that the selected subset is a representative of the whole population. In this chapter, we will learn about the commonly used sampling types and methods among allied health professionals. Examples have been for better understanding.

A. Hazari, *Research Methodology for Allied Health Professionals*,
https://doi.org/10.1007/978-981-99-8925-6_6

6.2 Need for Sampling

Sampling in research is a crucial step as it allows the researchers to be specific in their sample collection ensuring accuracy in the research methodology. It also helps to save time in selecting the desired sample through a systematic approach and finally the purpose of research, which is the application of results from a sample group to the entire population that is well met when the sampling procedure is correct. Therefore, sampling in the research holds a strong significance.

6.3 Sampling Types and Methods

There are two types of sampling, viz. probability sampling and non-probability sampling, and various subtypes are included in determining its sampling method as schematically represented in Fig. 6.1. We will try to learn its type and its method of application in detail with examples in various streams for allied health sciences.

6.4 Probability Sampling

As the name suggests, the sampling allows equal opportunity for each sample to be included with a known probability. Probability sampling is most appropriate for the homogenous group, where all samples share common characteristics and features;

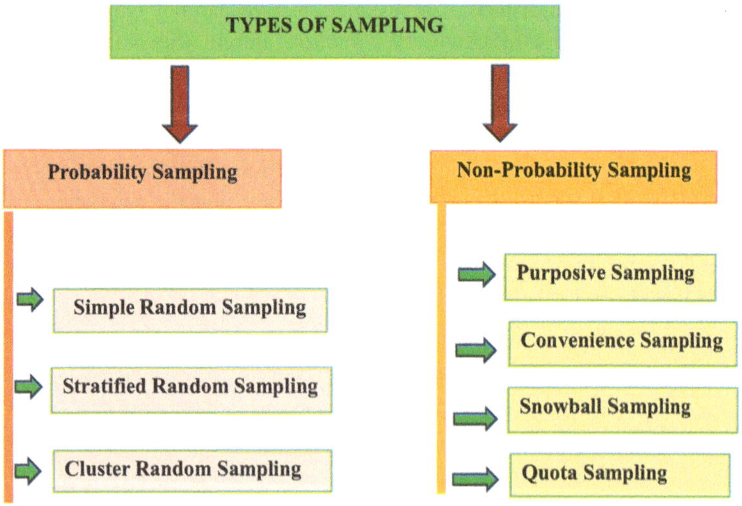

Fig. 6.1 Types and methods of sampling

therefore, selection of any sample has the same probability and would be considered as an ideal sample representative of the entire population. For example, a researcher wants to conduct a study on lung complications among Covid-19 patients. He has a list of 1000 Covid-19 patients (homogenous group), and he requires 100 samples for his study. He would use probability sampling for the selection of the sample population, where all 1000 participants would have a 100% chance of being selected. Probability sampling is most appropriately and widely used for experimental studies but can be applied to descriptive studies. A researcher may use the following methods for probability sampling based on the study objective, research design, and available resources for the desired study.

6.4.1 Simple Random Sampling

The random selection of participants in the study ensures the unbiased process of sample recruitment and data collection, which is the essence of probability sampling. In simple random sampling, researchers use a simple method of randomization such as the lottery method, tossing a coin, and chit system. This is to ensure that the selection of participants is under control of its probability of being either selected or not selected with an easy and simple method.

Example 6.1
A physical therapist wants to research low-level laser therapy and musculoskeletal conditions with the following research details.

Null hypothesis: There is no statistically significant effect of low-level laser therapy in ankle sprain.

Alternate hypothesis: There is a statistically significant effect of low-level laser therapy in ankle sprain.

Objective: To determine the efficacy of low-level laser therapy on pain among athletes with grade 2 ankle sprain

Sampling: The researcher would select an experimental research design and conduct a simple random sampling where he can use a paper chit to write "Yes" or "No" on a concealed envelope and ask the participant to choose one paper chit. This is a type of simple random sampling.

Example 6.2
A medical lab professional wants to conduct research on kidney functions among diabetics with the following research details:

Null hypothesis: There are no statistically significant changes in kidney functions among diabetic populations.

Alternate hypothesis: There are statistically significant changes in kidney functions among diabetic populations.

Objective: To determine the levels of bilirubin in the urine among type 2 diabetes mellitus patients

Sampling: The researcher would select a descriptive research design and conduct a simple random sampling where he can do a toss method to select or exclude participants. This would be a type of simple random sampling.

Example 6.3
A radio technician wants to research bone mineral density among young females with polycystic ovarian disorder with the following research details:

Null hypothesis: There is no statistically significant change in bone mineral density among young females with polycystic ovarian disorder.

Alternate hypothesis: There is a statistically significant change in bone mineral density among young females with polycystic ovarian disorder.

Objective: To determine the levels of calcium in long bones among young females with polycystic ovarian disorder using a DEXA scan.

Sampling: The researcher would select a descriptive research design and conduct a simple random sampling where he uses a random table of selected numbers (5, 10, 12, 17, 19 …) from 100 sample participants. This would be a type of simple random sampling.

Note: Lottery/chit, toss, and random tables are different techniques for conducting simple random sampling. One can also customize his/her way with the simple random method.

6.4.2 Stratified Random Sampling

This type of sampling includes a random selection of participants from a specified group called strata (group having similar characteristics) with lesser homogeneity as explained through examples below.

Example 6.4
A physical therapist wants to conduct a comparative study on the effects of aerobic training among diabetics, lung cancer survivors, and healthy participants.

Null hypothesis: There is no statistically significant difference in aerobic training among diabetics, lung cancer survivors, and healthy participants.

Alternate hypothesis: There is a statistically significant difference in aerobic training among diabetics, lung cancer survivors, and healthy participants.

Objective: To compare the peak Vo2 level among diabetics, lung cancer survivors, and healthy participants following 8 weeks of aerobic training program

Sampling: The researcher would select an experimental research design and first divide the participants into three different groups (strata), viz. diabetics, lung cancer survivors, and healthy from a pool of participants. Now, he would randomly select participants from each stratum to classify as strata random sampling method. It is possible that a participant could be diabetic as well as a lung cancer survivor, and thus homogeneity is diluted, which could be better dealt with strata random sampling.

Example 6.5
A medical laboratory professional would like to study the levels of HbA1C among diabetics with different blood groups (strata with blood group A, strata with blood group B, strata with blood group AB, strata with blood group O). The researchers would first stratify the diabetics as per their blood group type and then do random sampling. This would be known as strata sampling.

Steps to conduct strata random sampling:

- Firstly, choose and target the desired population.
- Identify stratification variables (age, height, disorder, religion, socioeconomic characteristics, etc.) matching with the research objective.
- Select the number of strata from the entire sample population as per the stated hypothesis and objective.
- Now use any simple random technique to finally select participants into the specified respective strata.

6.4.3 Systematic Random Sampling

When the data is huge, and the desired sample is required in a quick time, systematic random sampling could be the choice of action. It is an advanced form of simple random sampling, which systematically selects the sample as explained in the following example.

Example 6.6
A researcher wants to follow up on patients with physiotherapy treatment who have undergone ACL reconstruction over the last 3 years. He/she wanted to use the hospital medical record and found 10,000 eligible cases. The researcher wants to take 50% of cases as his/her sample. How would he/she select the sample?

He/she would need to conduct a systematic random sampling method, where he/she would assign numbers to all eligible patients and then every 7th number or 10th or Nth as per the choice of the researcher that could be selected through computer generation.

6.4.4 Cluster Random Sampling

Most of the researchers get confused between strata and cluster sampling; therefore, it would be good to first clarify the difference between the two. As discussed above, a stratum is a subgroup that we create from a homogenous group, whereas a cluster is a naturally defined group that can be either homogenous or heterogenous: for example, a cluster of people in a family, a cluster of people in a geographical region, and people in different religions. They are all naturally occurring groups sharing some similar or dissimilar characteristics.

Now let us try to understand the application of cluster random sampling in allied health streams with examples below.

Example 6.7

A physical therapist wants to conduct research on the effects of exercise in a specified program on youths of three different races, with the following research details:

Null hypothesis: There is no statistically significant difference in the effects of exercise based on race.

Alternate hypothesis: There is a statistically significant difference in the effects of exercise based on race.

Objective: To compare the effects of resistance training on young adults of Asian, Caucasian, and Arabic population

Sampling: The researcher would conduct an experimental study with participants in clusters of Asian, Caucasian, and Arabic regions following which a random sampling technique would be applied to select the sample.

Example 6.8

A medial laboratory researcher wants to identify the dietary habits affecting the blood sugar levels between Hindus, Muslims, and Christians. He/she would first choose a cluster of people in their respective religion and then perform random sampling to classify as a cluster random sampling method of probability sampling type.

Note: **"Multistage sampling"** is a complex form of cluster sampling, where samples are selected from clusters and sub-clusters at different stages.

6.5 Non-probability Sampling

This type of sampling does not require the process of randomization, and therefore the sample does not have a known probability of being selected or rejected; rather, it is direct recruitment of the desired sample from the population. The different methods of non-probability sampling have been discussed below with examples.

6.5.1 Purposive Sampling

As the name suggests, the sample is selected according to the purpose of the study and is also known as "deliberate sampling" or "judgmental sampling" since the decision to select the sample is both deliberate and based on judgment by the researcher. The study population is well defined to apply purposive sampling.

Example 6.9

A physical therapist wants to conduct a study to determine the knee joint power in footballers. Since it is clear to the researcher that he/she has to conduct the study among footballers, only footballers would be eligible to be samples and thus selected. Further inclusion and exclusion criteria would be applied to the selected footballers to finally recruit the sample, but since they were directly and deliberately chosen, it would be a purposive sampling method under the non-probability sampling type.

6.5.2 Convenience Sampling

Like purposive sampling, convenience sampling is also a type of direct sampling method with the added advantage of choosing samples that are convenient to the researcher. In the above example for purposive sampling, footballers are required to be selected, which can be done from any sports club, sports organization, regional team, international platform, etc. However, I am an allied health medical student and footballer meeting the inclusion criteria as samples from my university are convenient for selection. This can be an example of convenient sampling.

6.5.3 Snowball Sampling

Unlike purposive and convenience sampling, snowball sampling is an indirect non-probability sampling method where the desired sample is difficult to find. In medical fields, this type of sampling is used for rare diseases where one sample would draw the selection of the other sample through known contacts, family, referrals, etc.

Example 6.10
A researcher wants to study the physical activity levels of Covid-19 female survivor patients. He/she uses contact of a sample to draw other samples, which would be a type of snowball sampling.

Note: If a researcher finds contacts of other samples through a sample already recruited through purposive or convenient sampling, it would not be considered as snowball. Remember that snowball is for rare conditions where samples are difficult to contact directly.

6.5.4 Quota Sampling

A quota is a group of people with similar characteristics as the strata; however, a quota can contain both homogenous and heterogenous groups. This type of sampling can be considered reciprocal to stratified sampling or cluster sampling done without randomization. It would be well suited for descriptive studies.

Example 6.11
A physical therapist wants to observe the physical activity levels among females pre- and postpartum.

Null hypothesis: There is no statistically significant difference in the physical activity levels among females pre- and postpartum.

Objective: To determine the metabolic equivalent among females pre- and postpartum

Sampling: The researcher would conduct an observational study selecting the participants into two quotas of pregnancy and postdelivery, respectively, following which physical activity levels between the two would be compared.

6.6 Process of Advanced Randomization in Sampling: Block Randomization

We learned that probability sampling uses a randomization method for the selection of the sample; however, the simple random method could lead to certain difficulties where sampling is required for interventional studies within a specified timeframe. Let us understand this with the following example.

Example 6.12
An allied health master student wants to conduct a study to determine the effects of aerobic training compared to resistance training on cardiovascular endurance among elite running athletes for 8 weeks. He/she would need to first select a pool of elite running athletes and then do a simple random sampling to identify the groups labelled as "aerobic training intervention," "resistance training intervention," and "control" group, respectively. The researcher has been allotted a timeframe of 6 months for data recruitment. However, from a pool of eligible samples, uneven participants have gone into the respective group for the initial 3 months because of simple random sampling. Maximum samples got into one group using the lottery method: for instance, 17 in aerobics, 6 in resistance, and 3 in control. This is a serious problem for the researcher considering that the researcher requires 40 samples in each group within a timeframe of 6 months including 8 weeks of training.

This sort of issue in research sampling could be sorted using advanced randomization such as "block randomization." The researcher makes small blocks of samples under each group and then tries to fill the blocks one by one such that even distribution happens. For instance, in the example above, if the researcher makes blocks of 10×4 for each three groups, the problem of uneven sample distribution could be restricted in such a way that once a block in a group is filled, the sample would be put into the block of the other group.

6.7 Blinding in Sampling

The process of randomization leads to unbiasedness to a certain and significant extent, which could further be enhanced using the process of "blinding." It is possible that though the researcher has followed the randomization, he/she may consider allocating participants into a desired group to favor the research hypothesis. To combat this, blinding is done such that the researcher is unaware of the group allocation and sampling is performed by a third person not related to the study. Thus, the researcher is masked for the process of sampling. which is known as ***"single blinding."*** It is also a research practice where the sample/participants need to be masked in addition to the researcher to avoid any error in the data collection results, which would be known as ***"double blinding."*** For example, if the research study wants to know the perception of healthcare workers for providing additional benefits, participants should be blinded and unaware of the outcome so that they do not put the responses in anticipation of the benefits.

6.8 Summary

Sampling is an essential step in research methodology to ensure that the results of the study can be generalized to the population with higher levels of confidence and accuracy. It is also an essential process to avoid biases in the research.

Chapter 7
Review of Literature: Search Engines and Strategies

7.1 Background

The review of literature or literature review is a critical and comprehensive analysis of existing literature (published research, articles, books, and other sources) on a particular topic or research question. It serves multiple purposes, including identifying gaps in current knowledge, synthesizing relevant information, and providing context for new research. Review of literature is an important and separate section in research project proposals, theses, and dissertations. However, in the original research manuscript, the section is merged in the background and not separately given. The review of literature is most importantly used in systematic review studies. The review of literature starts with an introduction of the topic and its relevance. The scope and objectives of the review should be defined along with highlighting the key themes, concepts, and research questions. A researcher can follow the steps below to conduct a comprehensive review of the literature.

7.1.1 Identification of Search Engine and Strategy

This is the most important and first step for a comprehensive literature search. It is important to remember that researchers should not limit their search to a limited database. Often, students only search PubMed considering that the literature search is complete; however, they miss many published studies that may have been within the scope of their review of the literature. Thus, comprehensive literature should involve various databases through such engines as Scopus, Web of Science, PubMed/Medline, Cochrane, CINAHL, ScienceDirect, Springer, Pedro, SPORTDiscus, and Google Scholar.

A. Hazari, *Research Methodology for Allied Health Professionals*,
https://doi.org/10.1007/978-981-99-8925-6_7

Following the selection of databases and search engines, researchers should identify their keywords and use them to run a search engine. It is important to understand here that this keyword list should be as big as possible and not limited to what is required for research writing. The search engine has advanced functions for using your keywords. The ***Boolean operators*** allow the use of the keywords in a specific manner. We will learn how to conduct a literature search through the example below.

Example 7.1

An allied health student wants to conduct a literature search for his master's thesis. The student has identified his research area of interest and designed his hypothesis and objectives with the title is as follows:

Title: "Efficacy of Mulligan mobilization in low back pain among diabetes mellitus"

Task: Conduct a comprehensive literature search.

Step 1: Select wider databases and search engines as discussed above.

Step 2: Identify keywords and make keyword sets as follows:

- Keyword set 1: effect, Mulligan, low back, diabetes mellitus

Note: The Keyword set 1 is directly taken from the title and students often make a mistake of using the limited keywords from the title only. Remember that the purpose of literature search is to dig all the previous publications within the scope of your research. Therefore it is possible that different researchers would have worked and published on similar themes but with different keywords in their research title. For instance effectiveness could be used as "intervention" or "application." Thus the use of multiple keyword sets would be required. These keywords are selected by the researcher based on understanding and expertise in the subject. In this example, I have shown three sets of keywords. However a researcher can think of and use as many as numbers of keyword sets

- Keywords set 2: Application, mobilization, low back, pain, type 2 diabetes mellitus
- Keywords set 3: intervention Mulligan mobilization back pain T2DM

Step 3: Use of Booleans: The Booleans used in the literature search include AND/OR NOT and BOTH in major databases

- Use the Boolean "AND" to connect unrelated keywords such as mobilization AND low back: Low back AND pain, Mulligan AND pain, AND diabetes mellitus.
- Use the Boolean "OR" for keywords that could replace each other such as application OR intervention OR effectiveness.
- Use the Boolean "NOT" to specify and focus the search such as diabetes mellitus NOT gestation diabetes NOT type 1 diabetes mellitus.
- Use the Boolean "BOTH" where you wish to include a larger search through a single keyword such as T1DM T2DM "BOTH."

Let us conduct the above search example in PubMed for better understanding explained through the following pictorial representations using Keyword sets 1, 2, and 3.

Step 1: Go to the PubMed web page, and use the advanced search builder option (Fig. 7.1)

Step 2: Enter keywords using Boolean through the ADD section (Fig. 7.2). Check your keywords for correct use in the Query Box. You can also use the All Fields dropout for specific inclusion and exclusion of your search.

Step 3: Click on Search to yield the search results (Fig. 7.3). You could further use the filter option on the left side of the screen to further limit your search options under specific types of publication, date, year, etc.

Step 4: Save the search results into an Excel sheet (.CSV) using the save option for further screening (Fig. 7.4). You could also directly send the results to the citation manager.

Step 5: Repeat the process for other databases, and make a master Excel file for the screening process.

7.1.2 Screening of Search Data

The screening process of the search data is done after obtaining the total search results. The first step in the screening process is the removal of ***"Duplication"*** since the same article could be indexed in multiple databases. It is easy to conduct the duplicate removal task through the Excel file on the data tab; therefore, researchers often organize their search results into a single file from all databases. Following this, all search results are individually screened first for ***"Title Screening"*** followed by ***"Abstract Screening."*** Results that are not relevant to the scope of the review or contents that look different are removed. Now the final selection of results qualifies for full-text screening as per the defined inclusion and exclusion criteria for the review.

Note: The exclusion and exclusion criteria for the review of literature are predefined by the researcher but are applied at the time of full screening to obtain the final number of studies to be included in the review.

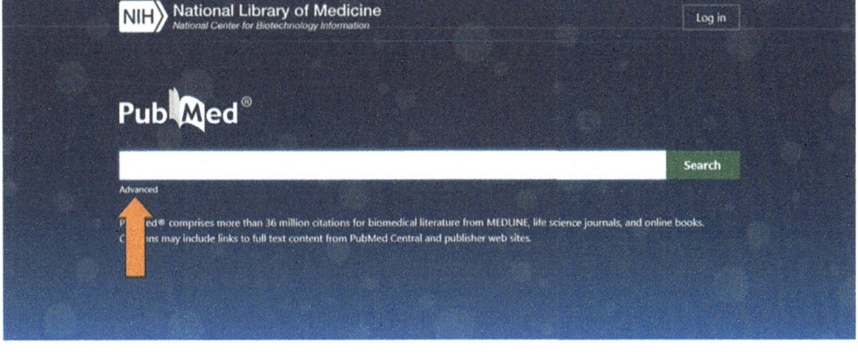

Fig. 7.1 Advanced search option in PubMed

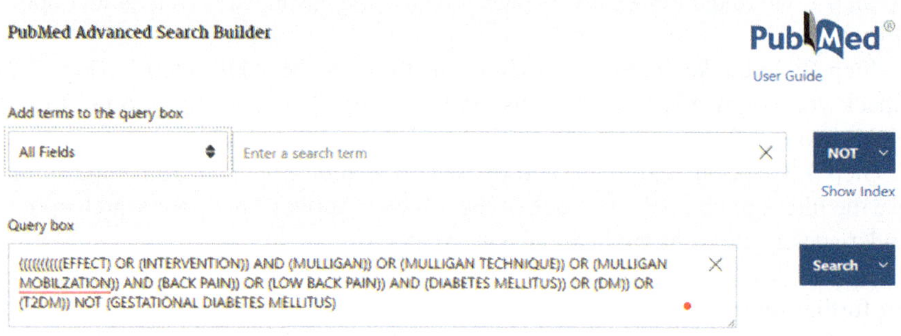

Fig. 7.2 The use of keywords and Boolean in PubMed

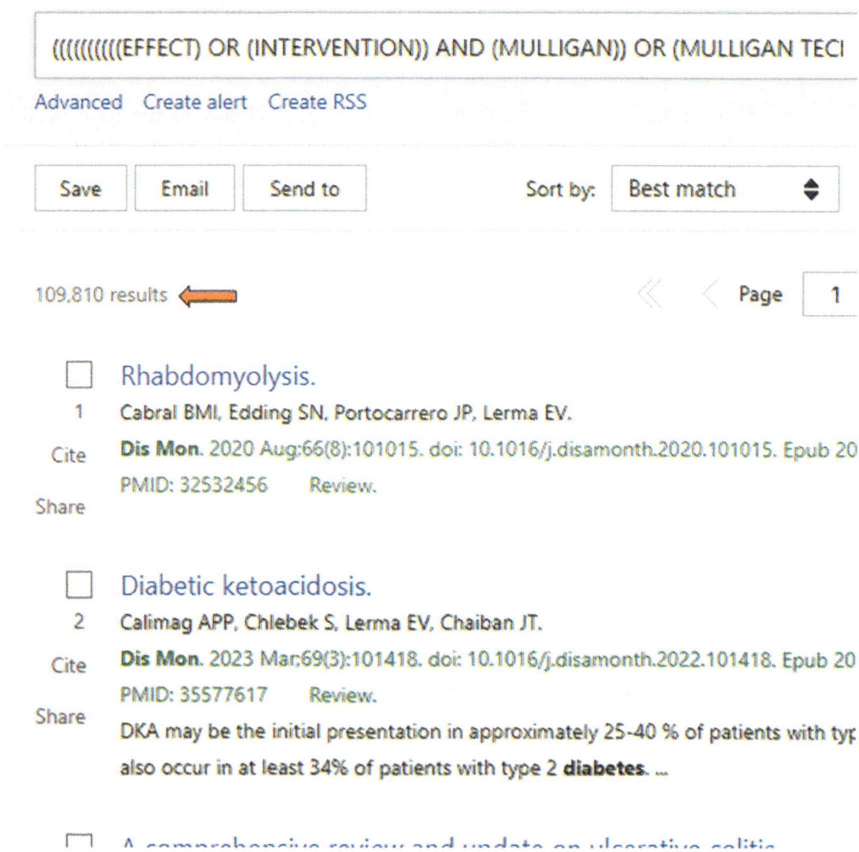

Fig. 7.3 The number of search results

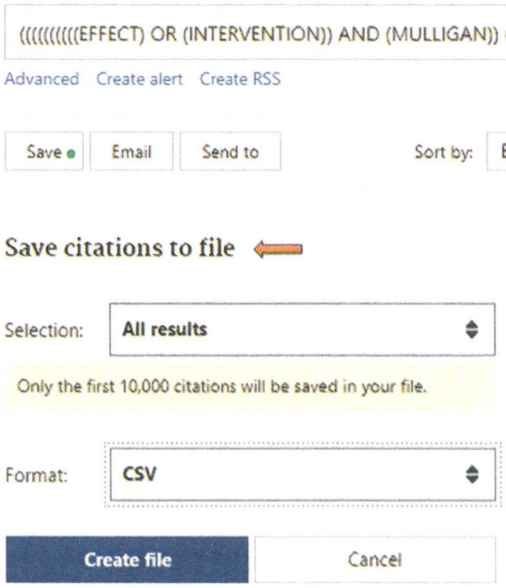

Fig. 7.4 Save option for searched results on PubMed

7.1.3 Data Reporting

The number of results at each stage should be carefully noted and reported as the search flow diagram. One of the most used templates is as described in the PRISMA statement for systematic review (Fig. 7.5) (Liberati et al. 2009) and review of published flow diagrams (Page et al. 2021).

7.1.4 Synthesis of Literature

After the data reporting, the synthesis or literature is done where reviewed articles are organized into themes or categories. It is important to summarize the main findings of each source and how they contribute to the overall understanding of the topic while also highlighting any contrasting viewpoints or areas of consensus among the sources.

7.1.5 Critique and Analysis

This involves evaluating the strengths and limitations of each source, considering factors like methodology, sample size, data analysis, and theoretical framework. The main purpose is to identify any biases or gaps in the existing literature. It would

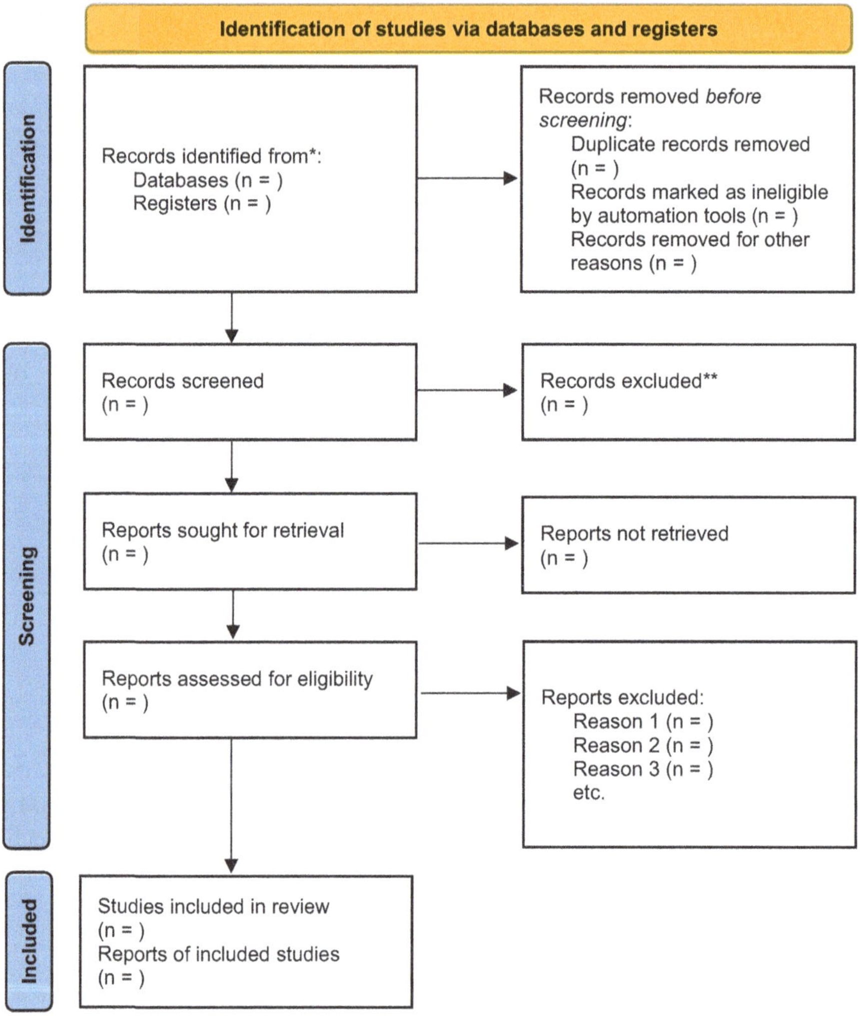

Fig. 7.5 Search flow diagram, PRISMA statement 2020 (Page et al. 2021)

be important to point out areas where the current literature lacks sufficient coverage or where contradictions exist and explain how these gaps are important and how they relate to your research question or objectives. Conducting a critical appraisal has been discussed separately in the upcoming chapters. An example of the synthesis of results (Table 7.1) and analysis of the review of literature of the Master of Physical Therapy thesis report has been given below. However, researchers could use their format of reporting.

Research Title: Comparison of Isokinetic Strength for Quadriceps and Hamstrings Among Recreational Athletes in UAE Playing Football, Cricket, and Tennis

Table 7.1 Worked out template for data synthesis from review of literature

S. No.	Title	Author and year	Methodology	Conclusion
1.	Plyometric-based Training for Isokinetic Knee Strength and Jump Performance in Cricket Fast Bowlers	Krishna et al. (2019)	42 professional fast bowlers were randomly assigned to a training group and a control group. Testing for isokinetic knee strength, vertical jump, and standing broad jump were performed on both groups. Functional H:Q ratio, BSAs, and DCRs were used as an outcome measure for ISE.	A significant improvement in jump performance and eccentric strength. The percentage of bowlers with poor BSA and DCR decreased. Plyometric training enhances dynamic knee strength in cricket fast bowlers, lowering injury risk and enhancing performance.
2.	Efficacy of Electromyographic-Biofeedback Supplementation Training with Patellar Taping on Quadriceps Strengthening in Patellofemoral Pain Syndrome Among Young Adult Male Athletes	Alonazi et al. (2021)	Sixty young adult male athletes with patellofemoral pain syndrome were randomly divided into EMG-BF-guided isometric exercise training with patellar taping and isometric exercise program along with EMG-BF. The Kujala Anterior Knee Pain Scale, the Visual Analog Scale, and the ISOMOVE Dynamometer were used to quantify quadriceps strength, functional impairment, and pain during the study's 4-week duration.	Four weeks of EMG-BF supplementation training with patellar taping demonstrated significant improvements in pain intensity, functional disability, and quadriceps muscle strength in young adult male athletes with PFPS.
3.	The Mechanism of Hamstring Injuries: A Systematic Review	Danielsson et al. (2020)	A systematic search was conducted using PubMed, Embase, and the Cochrane Library. The inclusion criteria for the article were the article with English language and consist of mechanism of HSI.	When the knee is extended and the hips are flexed to a great extent, the hamstrings can suffer a stretch-type injury. Immense strain on muscle during swing phase of running due to eccentric contraction is the most common reason for HSI.

(continued)

Table 7.1 (continued)

S. No.	Title	Author and year	Methodology	Conclusion
4.	Hamstring Injuries in Elite Gaelic Football: An 8-Year Investigation to Identify Injury Rates, Time-Loss Patterns and Players at Increased Risk	Roe et al. (2016)	38 datasets from 15 elite male Gaelic football teams were received by the National Gaelic Athletic Association (GAA) Injury Surveillance Database between 2008 and 2015. Data on injuries and exposure were made available online by the team's medical professionals.	HSI is the most frequent injury in elite Gaelic football, with incidences increasing from 2008–2011 to 2012–2015. The prevalence of HSI may be decreased by adjusting risk management tactics based on injury history, age, and playing position.
5.	Low Pre-season Hamstring-to-Quadriceps Strength Ratio Identified in Players Who Further Sustained In-Season Hamstring Strain Injuries: A Retrospective Study from a Brazilian Serie A Team	Veeck et al. (2023)	One professional football team from the Brazilian Serie A league participated in the study, who have completed a total of 4–5 football training sessions and 1–2 matches every week, and a total of 73 matches and 6570 min of match time throughout the season. Using a Biodex isokinetic dynamometer, the conventional and functional ratios were determined by recording the highest PTs of each muscle activity.	Pre-season H:Q ratios (conventional and functional ratios, CR and FR) were lower, and concentric PT was greater for injured players (IPs) than uninjured players (UPs), according to the findings. Furthermore, low FR and CR ratings were connected with high levels of quadriceps concentric PT, and individual data analysis revealed that this connection was stronger in the IP than in the UP. Athletes with in-season HSI showed higher concentric PT of quadriceps and lower FR and CR during pre-season than athletes with UP but no corresponding hamstring PT involving imbalance in strength due to increased H:Q resulting in higher probability towards injury.

S. No.	Title	Author and year	Methodology	Conclusion
6.	Rapid Hamstrings to Quadriceps Ratio at Long Muscle Lengths in Professional Football Players with Previous Hamstring Strain Injury	Correia et al. (2020)	24 professional male football players (12 with and 12 without previous HSI) performed maximal voluntary isometric contractions at long hamstring lengths and isokinetic concentric and eccentric contractions. On the basis of PT, CR and FR were calculated.	The hypothesis that a poor response to injury may be to blame for the somewhat lower early contraction (100 ms) RTD H:Q ratio seen in the previously damaged group. The study believes that if injury-related pain is left untreated, persistent inhibition may develop and compromise certain long hamstring lengths.
7.	Muscle Injuries in Athletes: The Relationship Between H/Q ratio (Hamstring/Quadriceps Ratio)		The purpose of the study was to investigate the association between the H:Q ratio and sprint timings and jump heights in football players. The study included 26 young top soccer players. Using a Cybex dynamometer, the PT was assessed.	It is noticeable that the asymmetries/imbalances in the FR have a direct link to the probability of the injury. According to published research, muscular imbalance might raise the risk factors for muscle injuries, particularly to the hamstring.
8.	Side-to-Side Asymmetry in Lower Limb Strength and Hamstring-Quadriceps Strength Ratio Among Collegiate American Football Players	Tatlıcıoğlu et al. (2019)	26 varsity American football players volunteered to undergo measurements of average PT for isokinetic flexion and extension of dominant limb and nondominant limb. H:Q ratio and limb asymmetry index were also calculated for both muscles.	To prevent possible lower limb injury and to increase performance, varsity American football players who are actively training and competing might consider taking strength asymmetry into account to tailor their strength training program accordingly.

(continued)

Table 7.1 (continued)

S. No.	Title	Author and year	Methodology	Conclusion
9.	The Association Between the Isokinetic Muscle Strength and Lower Extremity Injuries in Young Male Football Players	Namazi et al. (2019)	73 under-21 football players were assessed by the isokinetic system pro 4 for the ISE of the hip, knee, and ankle muscles.	According to the findings, lower limb injury incidence is highly influenced by hip and knee muscle strength mainly among football players and is related to isokinetic strength of lower limb muscles.
10.	The Effect of the "11+ Kids" Program on the Isokinetic Strength of Young Football Players	Zarei et al. (2020)	The control and intervention groups were allocated. Two days prior to and after the 10-week intervention, the ISE was performed.	There was an improvement and gain in strength in the intervention group, which improved performance of the players and resulted in a reduction of risk of injury.
11.	Using Isokinetic Strength Assessment to Predict Performance and Prevent Injuries in Indian Cricket Fast Bowlers	Krishna et al. (2019)	Pitchers were recruited. Proteus technology was used to measure throwing mechanics and isolated arm motions. A single set of biceps and triceps movements as well as a biomechanical assessment of a throwing movement were recorded.	Fast bowlers are more vulnerable to injury because of their unfavorable strength asymmetry and dynamic control ratio. Increasing dynamic knee strength with plyometric exercise may enhance performance and lower the risk of injury.

S. No.	Title	Author and year	Methodology	Conclusion
12.	Analysis Isokinetic Muscular Strength of Knee Flexors and Extensors Between Bowlers, Batsman and Wicketkeepers in Cricket	Das et al. (2020)	15 male university cricket players (5 bowlers, 5 batters, and 5 wicketkeepers) were purposefully chosen. The strength of the knee flexion and extension muscles was measured using an isokinetic dynamometer. To avoid injury, the individuals did adequate warming up of the lower leg muscles involved in the testing prior to the test. When the test began, the participant used maximal force to flex and extend the leg. The results were entered into a computer. The outcome was shown on the machine's monitor.	It may be established that the bowler, batter, and wicketkeeper all have equivalent knee flexor and knee extensor strength. As a result, coaches or physical trainers have to come up with a strength plan to increase lower limb muscles for improved performance and injury prevention.
13.	Are There Differences in Concentric Isokinetic Strength Performance Profiles Between International and Non-international Elite Soccer Players?	Śliwowski et al. (2021)	100 male soccer players were included in the cohort for this study, of whom 36 competed at the international level (IL) and 64 at the professional (non-international) elite level (N-IL). All athletes in the IL and N-IL categories had played professional football for at least 3 years and have been regularly trained. The research was done between 2010 and 2019. Every measurement was taken twice a year, at the start of the pre-season and the regular season. Each participant had two functional movement screen assessments, two proprioception tests, two isokinetic hamstring and quadriceps strength tests, and two ground response force analyses as part of their regular biomechanical evaluations during each season.	It suggests that variations in training adaptations and the degree of competitiveness among the players may be the cause of the intergroup variation in hamstring muscle strength. It follows logically that regular strength training of these muscle groups is highly advised since knee flexor strength is very significant in football players for repeated high-intensity bouts of exercise and for joint stabilization throughout varied jobs. Additionally, the study discovered H:Q ratio intergroup variations that were statistically significant.

(continued)

Table 7.1 (continued)

S. No.	Title	Author and year	Methodology	Conclusion
14.	Isokinetic Strength, Bilateral and Unilateral Strength Differences: Variation by Age and Laterality in Elite Youth Football Players	Maly et al. (2021)	70 elite male players are divided into four age groups from the same professional football team. In this study, body mass was determined using a digital scale, and height was determined using a digital stadiometer. ISE was performed with 90° knee flexion/ extension.	The study showed that 17-year-old players have levels of strength similar to under-19 players. The bilateral difference between knee flexors and extensors was found to be larger, indicating that knee flexors should be given more attention. For strength and strength asymmetries, there was no evidence of a laterality effect.
15.	Muscle Strength and Hamstrings to Quadriceps Ratio in Young Soccer Players: A Cross-Sectional Study	Mandroukas et al. (2023)	265 young soccer players were recruited for the study. Athletes between the ages of 12 and 14 had a 44-week training season, whereas those between the ages of 16 and 20 had a 46-week season. The CR was determined for each participant.	Training at a high intensity could improve the H:Q ratio, shielding the knee joint from heavy loads, suggesting that the H:Q strength ratio is low in younger people and substantial in elderly persons.
16.	Prediction of Hamstring Injury in Professional Soccer Players by Isokinetic Measurements	Dauty et al. (2016)	From 2001 to 2011, 350 isokinetic tests were performed in 136 professional soccer players at the beginning of the soccer season. Fifty-seven players suffered hamstring injury during the season that followed the isokinetic tests. These players were compared with the 79 uninjured players.	The prevalence of HSI varied by position on the field, with forwards having a greater incidence than midfielders, defenders, and goalkeepers. The chance of a hamstring injury in professional football players throughout the competitive season may be predicted using isokinetic ratios. It could be associated with various muscular strength profiles. In addition, soccer players would have muscular injuries more frequently during games than during training.

S. No.	Title	Author and year	Methodology	Conclusion
17.	Nordic Hamstring Strength of Highly Trained Youth Football Players and Its Relation to Sprint Performance	Markovic et al. (2020)	22 adult and 133 highly trained youth footballers in the age groups under (U)12–U18 participated in this study. Eccentric hamstring strength was assessed using the Nordic Hamstring (NH) device. Youth footballers also performed 20-m sprint test.	Both the absolute and relative NH strength increases with players' age; however, this increase was not linear and was the highest in U16 age group. The highest values were found in the U12 and U13 age groups, with nonsignificant variations in bilateral NH strength asymmetry (8–16%) between age groups. Finally, it was reported that relative NH strength might account for 27% of the variance in the sprint performance of young football players.

DCRs dynamic control ratios, *BSA* bilateral strength asymmetries, *NCAA* National Collegiate Athletic Association

The tabulated information could also be written in paragraphs as discussed below:

Krishna et al. (2019) figured out how the fast bowlers' isokinetic knee strength would be affected by a combination of plyometric and strength training programs. Bilateral strength asymmetries (BSAs), dynamic control ratios (DCRs), and eccentric and concentric PT in the quadriceps and hamstrings were all evaluated using isokinetic testing. The study concluded that eccentric strength and jump performance both significantly improved in 12 weeks, and reduced BSA and DCR scores were noted among the bowlers. In cricket fast bowlers, enhancing dynamic knee strength with plyometric exercise minimizes the risk of injuries and increases performance.

Alonazi et al. (2021) conducted a study to evaluate the advantages of isometric exercise alone versus isometric training assisted by electromyographic-biofeedback (EMG-BF) in young adult male athletes with patellofemoral pain syndrome (PFPS). Participants followed their various fitness regimens 5 days a week for a total of 4 weeks. The findings of the study were evaluated using the Visual Analog Scale for pain, the Kujala Anterior Knee Pain Scale for functional impairment, and the ISOMOVE dynamometer for quadriceps strength. Four weeks of EMG-BF supplementation training in combination with patellar tape significantly reduced pain intensity, functional impairment, and strength of quadriceps muscles in young adult male athletes with PFPS.

Danielsson et al. (2020) analyzed the mechanism of hamstring strain injury (HSI), which is the most common in sports and results in significant time loss. The results of this study indicate that persistent hip flexion with an extended knee causes stretch-type hamstring strain. The most frequent factor contributing to HSI during sprinting is excessive muscle stress brought on by eccentric contraction during the late swing phase of the running gait cycle.

Roe et al. (2016) in their study collected 38 datasets from 15 premier male Gaelic football teams between 2008 and 2015 and revealed that HSI is the most common with rates rising from 2008 to 2011; therefore, to reduce the incidence of HSI, adjusting risk management tactics according to injury history, age, and playing position should be employed.

Mandroukas et al. (2023) on young soccer players assessed the concentric isokinetic PT of the knee flexors and extensors and compared their ratio. The study's findings suggest that vigorous exercise may improve the H:Q strength ratio, which in turn protects the knee joint against large loads. This is because the H:Q strength ratio is low in youth and high in old age.

According to Veeck et al. (2023), in their study, players who suffered HSI during a season for a professional South American football team were those who had lower pre-season H:Q functional ratio and conventional ratios. It may be possible to reduce the incidence of in-season in the squad by using resistance training techniques that promote an equal H:Q strength balance and proportionate muscle activation patterns for dynamic knee joint stability.

Paulo Correiato et al. (2020) in football players with and without prior HSI evaluated the rate of torque development (RTD) H:Q at long hamstring lengths, conventional (concentric/concentric) and functional (eccentric/concentric) H:Q ratios, and concluded that previously damaged hamstrings had minimal impacts on RTD H:Q and flexor eccentric torque. In late time intervals, the previous HSI group had a slight to moderately higher RTD H:Q.

Bhatt et al. intended the study to draw a connection between the hamstring and quadriceps' conventional and functional relationship and the rise in severe sports injuries, particularly muscular injuries. Muscle damage has been more common in recent years, according to scientific research. It has been found that the functional H:Q relationship's asymmetries and imbalances have a significant impact on the occurrence of muscle injury. Muscle imbalance has been linked to an increase in the risk factors for muscle injuries, particularly in the hamstring.

Tatlıcıoğlu et al. (2019) conducted a study on 26 American football players for the traditional H:Q ratio and the limb asymmetry index as risk factors for lower limb injuries. The results demonstrated that players who are actively training and competing should consider a strength training program for strength asymmetry to improve performance.

Śliwowski et al. (2021) concluded that there may be differences in training adaptations and degree of competition among the players, which may be the cause of intergroup variability in terms of hamstring muscle strength. Regular strength training of these muscle groups is highly advised because knee flexor strength is incredibly significant in soccer players for sustained high-intensity activity and for joint stabilization during diverse tasks. Additionally, the study discovered statistically significant intergroup variations in H:Q ratios. Greater performance and strength balance around the knee joint, as well as a higher potential for muscular joint stabilization, may be indicated by international players having this indicator at a higher level than non-international players, along with a greater reciprocal ratio and stronger hamstring muscles.

Markovic et al. (2020) conducted a study that comprised highly skilled under (U)-12–U18 football players and demonstrated that players' Nordic hamstring (NH) strength increased with age in both the absolute and relative senses; however, this gain was not linear and was maximum in the U16 age group. The age groups' differences in bilateral NH strength asymmetries were not statistically different, with the U12 and U13 age groups showing the greatest values. Finally, the study showed that certain variations in young football players' sprint performance might be attributed to relative NH strength.

Namazi et al. (2019) conducted a study to assess the risk of lower extremity injuries. According to the findings, lower limb injury incidence is highly influenced by hip and knee muscle strength, and lower limb injury incidence among football players is related to isokinetic strength of lower limb muscles. In addition, given the prevalence of ankle injuries, ankle function and damage are influenced by the strength of the knee and hip muscles. Therefore, research on the ISE ratio of the hip adductor/abductor, isokinetic strength of the hip abductor/adductor muscles, and isokinetic strength ratio of the knee flexor/extensor muscles can help raise awareness about the factors that lead to football injuries, consequently resulting in the emergence of a screening test to determine and prevent sports injuries.

7.1.6 Summary

The review of literature is one of the most essential sections of research methodology which helps to identify the existing gaps and allows researchers to plan their research hypothesis with a scientific base and support. For the thesis and dissertation, the review of the literature should be given in detail. Researchers are free to represent the findings with their ideas. The literature search strategy should be scientifically performed to ensure that all previous literature has been included for screening as per the inclusion and exclusion criteria.

References

Alonazi, A., Hasan, S., Anwer, S., Jamal, A., Parvez, S., Alfaiz, F.A.S. and Li, H., 2021. Efficacy of electromyographic-biofeedback supplementation training with patellar taping on quadriceps strengthening in patellofemoral pain syndrome among young adult male athletes. International journal of environmental research and public health, 18(9), p.4514.

Correia, P., Santos, P., Mil-Homens, P., Gomes, M., Dias, A. and Valamatos, M.J., 2020. Rapid hamstrings to quadriceps ratio at long muscle lengths in professional football players with previous hamstring strain injury. European Journal of Sport Science, 20(10), pp.1405–1413.

Danielsson, A., Horvath, A., Senorski, C., Alentorn-Geli, E., Garrett, W.E., Cugat, R., Samuelsson, K. and Hamrin Senorski, E., 2020. The mechanism of hamstring injuries–a systematic review. BMC musculoskeletal disorders, 21, pp.1–21.

Das, R., Jhajharia, B. and Kumar, D., 2020. Analysis isokinetic muscular strength of knee flexors and extensors between bowlers, batsman and wicketkeepers in cricket. Journal of Sports Science and Nutrition, 1(2), pp.50–53.

Dauty, M., Menu, P., Fouasson-Chailloux, A., Ferréol, S. and Dubois, C., 2016. Prediction of hamstring injury in professional soccer players by isokinetic measurements. Muscles, ligaments and tendons journal, 6(1), p.116.

Krishna, S.A., Alwar, T.K., Ramasamy, R., Vinayagam, S. and Sivaraman, A., 2019. Using Isokinetic Strength Assessment to Predict Performance and Prevent Injuries in Indian Cricket Fast Bowlers.

Krishna, S.A., Alwar, T.K., Sibeko, S., Ranjit, S. and Sivaraman, A., 2019. Plyometric-based training for isokinetic knee strength and jump performance in cricket fast bowlers. International journal of sports medicine, 40(11), pp.704–710.

Liberati A, Altman DG, Tetzlaff J, Mulrow C, Gøtzsche PC, Ioannidis JP, Clarke M, Devereaux PJ, Kleijnen J, Moher D. The PRISMA statement for reporting systematic reviews and meta-analyses of studies that evaluate healthcare interventions: explanation and elaboration. BMJ. 2009 Jul 21;339:b2700. doi: https://doi.org/10.1136/bmj.b2700. PMID: 19622552; PMCID: PMC2714672.

Maly, T., Ford, K.R., Sugimoto, D., Izovska, J., Bujnovsky, D., Hank, M., Cabell, L. and Zahalka, F., 2021. Isokinetic Strength, Bilateral and Unilateral Strength Differences: Variation by Age and Laterality in Elite Youth Football Players. International Journal of Morphology, 39(1).

Mandroukas, A., Michailidis, Y. and Metaxas, T., 2023. Muscle Strength and Hamstrings to Quadriceps Ratio in Young Soccer Players: A Cross-Sectional Study. Journal of Functional Morphology and Kinesiology, 8(2), p.70.

Markovic, G., Sarabon, N., Boban, F., Zoric, I., Jelcic, M., Sos, K. and Scappaticci, M., 2020. Nordic hamstring strength of highly trained youth football players and its relation to sprint performance. The Journal of Strength & Conditioning Research, 34(3), pp.800–807.

Namazi, P., Zarei, M., Hovanloo, F. and Abbasi, H., 2019. The association between the isokinetic muscle strength and lower extremity injuries in young male football players. Physical therapy in sport, 39, pp.76–81.

Padasala, M., Joksimovic, M., Bruno, C., Melino, D. and Manzi, V., 2020. Muscle injuries in athletes. The relationship between H/Q ratio (hamstring/quadriceps ratio). Ita J Sports Reh Po, 7(1), pp.1478–1498.

Page MJ, McKenzie JE, Bossuyt PM, Boutron I, Hoffmann TC, Mulrow CD, et al. (2021) The PRISMA 2020 statement: An updated guideline for reporting systematic reviews. PLoS Med 18(3): e1003583.

Roe, M., Murphy, J.C., Gissane, C. and Blake, C., 2016. Hamstring injuries in elite Gaelic football: an 8-year investigation to identify injury rates, time-loss patterns and players at increased risk. British journal of sports medicine.

Śliwowski, R., Marynowicz, J., Grygorowicz, M., Wieczorek, A. and Jadczak, Ł., 2021. Are there differences in concentric isokinetic strength perfor-mance profiles between international and non-international elite soccer players?. International Journal of Environmental Research and Public Health, 18(1), p.35.

Tatlıcıoğlu, E., Atalağ, O., Kırmızıgil, B., Kurt, C. and Acar, M.F., 2019. Side-to-side asymmetry in lower limb strength and hamstring-quadriceps strength ratio among collegiate American football players. Journal of physical therapy science, 31(11), pp.884–888.

Veeck, F., Ruas, C.V., Pinto, M.D., Grazioli, R., Cardoso, G.P., Albuquerque, T., Schipper, L., Valente, H.G., Santos, V.H., Dornelles, M. and Rabaldo, P., 2023. Low pre-season hamstring-to-quadriceps strength ratio identified in players who further sustained in-season hamstring strain injuries: a retrospective study from a Brazilian Serie A team. Sports, 11(4), p.89.

Zarei, M., Abbasi, H., Daneshjoo, A., Gheitasi, M., Johari, K., Faude, O., Rommers, N. and Rössler, R., 2020. The effect of the "11+ kids" program on the isokinetic strength of young football players. International Journal of Sports Physiology and Performance, 15(1), pp.25–30.

Chapter 8
Developing Research Proposal

8.1 Background

A researcher most often gets stuck while writing a research proposal, as one may face common difficulties in how to start and end. It would be advisable for all readers to go through the previous chapters to understand the research terminology well. In this chapter, we will learn how to design a research proposal using the essential components of research methodology, which may apply to all allied health streams. These sections are essential for any research project and need to be listed in order. The same components would be sequentially used for all types of scientific research writing such as research proposals, research theses, dissertations, and research grant projects. Therefore, it would be very useful for all readers to first understand the components and their salient features and then use it for the requisite research purposes accordingly. Examples of different allied health streams have also been given for better understanding.

8.1.1 Title of the Research Project

The first and foremost component of any research project is the "title." The title of any research project could be considered as the outer covering of the project representing what is present inside. Thus, the entire research project could be well reflected with an appropriate title. In simple words, the title of the study can give the most valuable information about the hypothesis, type of study, population on which it is conducted, research methods, and predictable results, which emphasizes the need to design an appropriate research title. A good title should be short and informative and concisely highlight the details of the study being undertaken. If a title is well designed, one can easily predict the hypothesis, aim, and research methods

A. Hazari, *Research Methodology for Allied Health Professionals*,
https://doi.org/10.1007/978-981-99-8925-6_8

used in the study. A research title needs to synch with the other components of a research project.

Example 8.1
A physical therapist wants to conduct a study on the effects of aerobic training on cardiopulmonary endurance in the diabetic population. What could be an appropriate title? Multiple options could be thought over; a few examples are given here:

(a) *Effects of 12 weeks' aerobic training on cardiopulmonary endurance among diabetes mellitus.*
(b) *Aerobic training for cardiovascular endurance among diabetes mellitus in the MENA region: An experimental study*—in addition to the above, this title also gives information about where the study is supposed to be or being conducted, and what type of study design (experimental) would be used.
(c) *Association of 12 weeks' aerobic training and cardiovascular endurance among type 2 diabetes mellitus in the United Arab Emirates using spirometry: A randomized controlled trial*—this title is more informative than the two above as it additionally provides the following information which could help to define the research project with more clarity in the first instance.

- *12 weeks signifies the duration of the intervention.*
- *Spirometry: outcome measure that would give VO_2 max/peak VO_2 as the outcome variable.*
- *Association: statistical analysis used in the study to establish the relation between aerobic training and cardiovascular endurance.*
- *Randomized controlled trial: represents study design that is not only experimental but also suggests that at least two different groups would be present, i.e., experimental and control.*

Example 8.2
A medical laboratory technologist wants to conduct a study to determine the effects of Glycomet on kidney function. What could be an appropriate title? Multiple options could be thought over; a few examples are given here like above to best represent the research project:

(a) *Effect of Glycomet on the kidney function among diabetics.*
(b) *Correlation of Glycomet 500 mg and insulin glargine (Gla-100) with SGOT and SGPT levels among type 2 diabetes mellitus for 8 weeks: A randomized controlled trial*—this title has the following advantages and can help predict the research project much better without the need to read it full.

- *The dose of the intervention is given.*
- *The outcome variable like SGOT and SGPT is given, which could also help to predict the standard outcome measure.*
- *The correlation suggests that an association would be statistically established with Glycomet and insulin with kidney function test markers, respectively.*

- *Randomized controlled trial suggests that it is an experimental study with three groups involved, i.e.; experimental (Glycomet 500 mg), experimental (Gla-100), and controlled group.*

Example 8.3
A radio technician wants to understand how gaming can affect the functions of the brain. What could be an appropriate title? Multiple options could be thought over; a couple of examples are given here like above to best represent the research project:

(a) *Gamification and brain function*—general title
(b) *Effects of 10 weeks' gamification on grey matter using anisotropy medical resonance imaging among stroke survivors*—specific title with more detailed information

Notes:

1. Some research proposals could also include a "running title," which is less descriptive and shorter, not more than 80–100 characters.
2. Avoid writing titles that are too lengthy and as paragraphs.

8.1.2 Introduction of the Research Project

The introduction of the research sets the theme of the research and is one of the most important components. The introduction section of any research proposal highlights the significance and the purpose of the study. It should be written in such a way that the topic chosen is worth selecting and has a significant impact. The introduction essentially includes a well-documented **statement of the problem/need of the study**, which forms the basis of the study to be proposed/conducted and clarifies the possible causes, knowledge gaps, and solution to the problem.

To start with the introduction, it is advisable to organize the available information to present the more general aspects of the topic to set up the background of the study, and then narrow it down to more specific contextual information in the middle section. Towards the end, one should ensure to provide existing lacunae in the current status of knowledge and state the **hypothesis** of the study followed by clear **aims and objectives.**

The **rationale** of the study is most often given separately to justify its uniqueness and predicted contribution to the research community.

Notes:

1. The introduction section in most of the research proposals has word limits (500–1000 words). Therefore, the researcher needs to organize all the essential information in a precise manner according to the word limit range.
2. There may be substantial changes in the subsection under the introduction according to the type of research proposal, but essential components remain the same as discussed above.

3. Citation should be done within the text as per the prescribed referencing format.
4. Some research proposals may require ***"Operational Definition"*** under the introduction section. The operational definition is given as a deviation from the standard definition if any as per the requirement in your study. For example, if you have included diabetes mellitus patients in your study and you wish to only include participants within the random blood sugar range of 120–140, you would be required to give an operational definition. In easy terms, operational definition allows you to customize your inclusion criteria where difficulty is faced to follow the standard definition.

8.1.2.1 Example: Writing Research Proposal Introduction for Physical Therapy Project—Word Limit 500–600

Title: Badminton for Cardiovascular and Neuromuscular Function Among Older Adults with and Without Noncommunicable Disease in the United Arab Emirates

Introduction: The success of well-being has been attributed to the higher level of physical activities in our day-to-day routine activities. The true meaning of fitness for humankind has a wider spectrum. It can be correlated with being free from various disorders including cardiovascular, musculoskeletal, neurological, and psychosocial conditions, and thus lead to an enhanced quality of life, which can be significantly achieved by incorporating adequate physical activities. The World Health Organization has declared physical inactivity as the fourth leading cause of death and a major risk factor for noncommunicable diseases. Physical activity can not only reverse the course of noncommunicable diseases but also prevent the progression of disease. Research from a variety of scientific fields suggests that physical activity in nature and feelings of connection to nature enhance psychological health and well-being (Lawton et al. 2017). Outdoor physical activity has higher benefits in lowering the levels of stress, anxiety, depression, and parameters related to noncommunicable diseases. It is well known that the presence of noncommunicable disease has a higher correlation with morbidity related to cardiovascular disorders, and aerobic training directly reflects the cardiovascular fitness of an individual. Given that adherence to physical activities is poor among older adults (>56 years) in the form of general aerobic training, engaging them in outdoor sports activities could be more useful to dampen the course of the noncommunicable disorders as well as prevent future complications. In addition, older adults are the most susceptible age group for developing neuromuscular and psychosocial disorders due to a lack of physical activity (Wilkinson et al. 2018). Loss of muscle strength, muscle tightness, reduced agility, poor balance and coordination, hand-eye coordination, etc. are very commonly seen as factors of reduced physical activity among older adults (Hunter et al. 2016) in addition to aging effects. Literature also suggests that the ill effects of aging can also be controlled with physical activity promotion (Cole et al. 2009).

Sports play a significant role in the promotion of physical activity. Badminton holds a significant position in popularity for outdoor sports. Among all sports, badminton targets the cardiovascular, musculoskeletal, and neurological systems significantly. The game requires constant engagement of the individual, which also improves their psychological and mental abilities and makes them more social. The noncontact nature of the sport makes it safer and suitable for any age group. The gender-friendly nature of sports, which is also widely accepted by various age groups, allows using it as a priority sport to enhance physical activity in research. Research has suggested that badminton puts significant demands on the cardiovascular and neuromuscular systems. The cardiovascular fitness parameter can be assessed by analyzing the VO_2 max capacity and expected as the primary outcome. Thus, the purpose of the study is to analyze the effects and promote physical activity using badminton sports on the physiological, biomechanical, and psychosocial changes among older adults (with and without noncommunicable diseases) of the United Arab Emirates (UAE).

Research Objectives

1. To analyze the changes in cardiovascular and neuromuscular fitness parameters for older adults with noncommunicable diseases in the UAE
2. To compare the changes in cardiovascular and neuromuscular fitness between older adults with and without noncommunicable disease while engaging in physical activity through badminton sport

Rationale/Need of the Study

Previous studies suggest that the higher prevalence of noncommunicable diseases adds to extreme health and financial burden to the United Arab Emirates, and promotion of physical activities could help combat this situation (Wilkinson et al. 2018). Thus, the project aims to reduce the burden of noncommunicable diseases by promoting outdoor physical activity while utilizing the beneficial effects of badminton sports on the physiological, biomechanical, and psychosocial aspects of humans.

8.1.2.2 Example: Writing Research Proposal Introduction for Medical Lab Project—Word Limit 200–300

Title: The prevalence of food poisoning by salmonella in the UAE

Introduction: In 2019, about 800 cases of food poisoning were reported in Dubai, and 150 restaurants were closed because of poor hygiene practices. Salmonella is an infection of the gastrointestinal tract. It is spread from person to person by the fecal-oral pathway, which occurs when an infected or asymptomatic person with poor hand or body cleanliness transfers the virus on to another person when handling food and water. Symptoms appear somewhere between 6 h and 6 days following infection. They include bloody diarrhea, a fever, and stomach cramps. Without antibiotic treatment, most patients recover in 4–7 days. However, some people with severe diarrhea may require hospitalization or antibiotic treatment. Salmonella germs can enter the bloodstream and migrate to the liver, kidneys, and other organs in severe situations. Antibiotics must be given to the person if this occurs. The infection might be fatal if treatment is not started as soon as possible. Salmonella can be controlled when people practice handwashing, good cooking, and storage temperature and avoid unpasteurized milk. The goal of the study is to determine the number of cases of salmonellosis in the United Arab Emirates.

Research Question and Hypothesis

What is the number of cases of salmonellosis in the UAE?

The null hypothesis of the study is that there is no significant prevalence of salmonellosis in the UAE.

The alternate hypothesis of the study is that there is a significant prevalence of salmonellosis in the UAE.

Objective: To determine the prevalence rate of salmonellosis in the UAE

8.1.2.3 Example: Writing Research Proposal Introduction for Anesthesia Technology—Word Limit 1000–1500

Title: The Effectiveness of Using Capnography for Early Detection of Hypoxemia During Endoscopic Sedation Monitoring in the Operating Theatre

Introduction: Hypoxemia continues to be a challenge in the field of gastrointestinal (GI) endoscopy. The common underlying mechanism of hypoxemia is insufficient ventilation induced by either hypoventilation or airway obstruction, which contributes to morbidity and death. Oxygen saturation (SaO_2) is a measurement of the percentage of oxygen transported by hemoglobin that may be determined reliably with a pulse oximeter. Currently, the pulse oximeter is being used to accurately measure oxygen saturation during endoscopy procedures. However, the use of a pulse oximeter only determines hypoxemia as it is happening but cannot early detect hypoxemia.

The detection of CO_2 in respiratory gases using capnography has become an essential component of anesthetic monitoring. A waveform is formed by measuring the carbon dioxide the patient exhales. Capnography monitoring is said to be more sensitive than current clinical routine monitoring of pulse oxygen saturation in identifying respiratory depression before the beginning of hypoxia as capnography shows a monitoring value as the patient exhales. There is a study conducted that states that capnography monitoring devices identify respiratory depression early on, therefore reducing the occurrence of hypoxemia in endoscopic procedures.

The purpose of this study is to find out if capnography can be utilized as a tool for the early detection of endoscopic procedure-related hypoxemia. This research aims to determine whether capnography monitoring is an effective tool to be used to early detect hypoxemia in operation theatres.

Need of the Study

A recent prospective study demonstrated how respiratory irregularities like apnea and hypoventilation frequently arise during colonoscopies carried out under sedation. Compared to the traditional use of pulse oximetry, capnography was simultaneously able to detect 38% of these anomalies more thoroughly and earlier by an average of 38.6 s. This is because the device capnography works by assessing the patient's carbon dioxide end-tidal volume, which is more sensitive to alveolar hypoventilation as opposed to oxygen saturation. Clinically, episodes of hypoxemia usually occur without any detectable signs in the patient's oxygen saturation levels through a pulse oximeter or evidence of mucosal color shift. This result is not unexpected given that the indications of hypoxemia frequently do not surface immediately until very low and dangerous levels of oxygen saturation develop. Although pulse oximetry is considered to be a sensitive test for the detection of hypoxemia, it is not the earliest and clear indicator of possible fatal airway issues since hypoxia is a relatively late sign of airway accidents and drops in oxygen levels prominently reflect desaturation. On the other hand, capnography is useful for spontaneously breathing and non-intubated patients. If oxygen is delivered simultaneously, these patients are prone to suffer respiratory depression and/or airway obstruction, which the pulse oximetry finds difficult to identify. Following that, evidence-based medicine describes how capnographic monitoring outperformed routine patient monitoring in detecting apnea and predicting oxygen desaturation during percutaneous transhepatic cholangiodrainage sedation.

Hence, following the points, revelations, effects, and patient safety concerns these studies have proved and highlighted, we are conducting this research to discover, identify, and study the effectiveness of using capnography for early detection of hypoxemia during endoscopic sedation monitoring.

Problem Statement

Pulse oximetry is typically the gold standard for accurately assessing the level of oxygen saturation in patients; however, it is unable to detect early warning signs of apnea, hypoventilation, or airway obstruction. Evidence-based studies promote the idea that capnography provides a superior method of assessing the ventilatory status of patients in comparison to pulse oximetry.

Objectives

Primary Objective

To determine the efficacy of capnography in the early detection of hypoxemia during endoscopic sedation monitoring in operation theatres

8.1.3 Research Methods

This section provides detailed information about where and how the study would be conducted keeping the scientific rigor in context to a selection of subjects, data collection procedure, data analysis, and ethical standards. Most of the research proposals would require filling the following sections under the methods heading.

8.1.3.1 Research Approach

Mention whether a qualitative or quantitative approach would be taken.

8.1.3.2 Research Design

Mention under the observational or experimental research design and their subtypes.

8.1.3.3 Research Setting

Place, institution, and center where the data collection would take place. It can be single-centered or multicentric, which needs to be mentioned in either case.

8.1.3.4 Ethical Approval and Issues

Here, the approval status of the research ethics committee needs to be mentioned along with the registration number if applied beforehand. In other cases, a statement suggesting that ethical approval from the concerned committee would be secured before data collection must be there. Also, any anticipated ethical concerns or issues need to be reported.

8.1.3.5 Sample Population (Inclusion and Exclusion Criteria)

The participants on which the research would be done need to be clearly defined along with the inclusion and exclusion criteria. It is important to understand the points written under the inclusion criteria that make it obvious to apply to the exclusion criteria and thus need not be mentioned in both. For example, if the inclusion criterion for age is 50–70 years, then there is no need to mention below 50 years and above upto 70 years as exclusion criteria as it is well understood and defined through inclusion itself.

8.1.3.6 Sample Size Calculation

The sample size needs to be mentioned in exact numbers along with the statistical tools and methods used to obtain it. The total sample size needs to be separately mentioned adding the dropout (usually 20%) for experimental studies with follow-up and nonrespondent rate of 15–20% for survey studies.

8.1.3.7 Sampling Method

Need to mention whether probability or non-probability type of sampling method would be taken for data recruitment. It is important to use the correct sampling method according to the study design. For instance, for experimental studies with control groups, a random sampling technique should be employed, or else it would lead to bias.

8.1.3.8 Outcome Variables and Outcome Measures

The primary and secondary outcome variables should be mentioned along with the outcome measure/tool to obtain the variables. For example, if one wishes to find the knee joint angle for a footballer while kicking a ball, the outcome variable would be the joint range of motion and the outcome variable could be goniometer or motion analysis system. Instead, if the objective is to determine the elbow joint muscle strength, then the variable could be joint power assessed by an isokinetic device as the outcome measure. The validity and reliability of the outcome measure from previously reported studies are usually mentioned in all research proposals.

8.1.3.9 Data Collection Procedure

This is the most important part of the research procedure and requires utmost attention for its accuracy. The procedure of conducting the research in a step-by-step sequential manner needs to be documented here. One can use the flowchart presentation to illustrate the necessary steps as shown in Fig. 8.1 for the study titled "Badminton for Cardiovascular and Neuromuscular Function Among Older Adults with and Without Noncommunicable Disease in the United Arab Emirates." Following sequential step actions, one also needs to describe in detail the standard procedure for collecting the data from all participants, which should not vary from subject to subject. For example, one physical therapist wants to check the effectiveness of ACL rehabilitation exercises on knee joint muscle strength after 6 weeks of training. He needs to give a standard protocol for ACL rehabilitation to all subjects (same exercise, same technique, same time duration, same room, same bed, under same environmental condition, etc.) as any deviation would lead to falsification of results.

Notes

1. Correct research methods and procedure are the backbone of any research. Efforts should be made to ensure the maximum accuracy of the data collection procedure and minimize bias in results.
2. At any point in time if an error in the research procedure is noted, the data should be removed from data analysis and interpretation and correct methodology should be employed for recollection of data.
3. The research methods section needs to be elaborate, and thus word limit is higher up to 1000–1500 words.

8.1.3.10 Research Timeline

All research proposals need to have a fixed and specified timeline. The use of a graphical representation or Gantt chart could be useful.

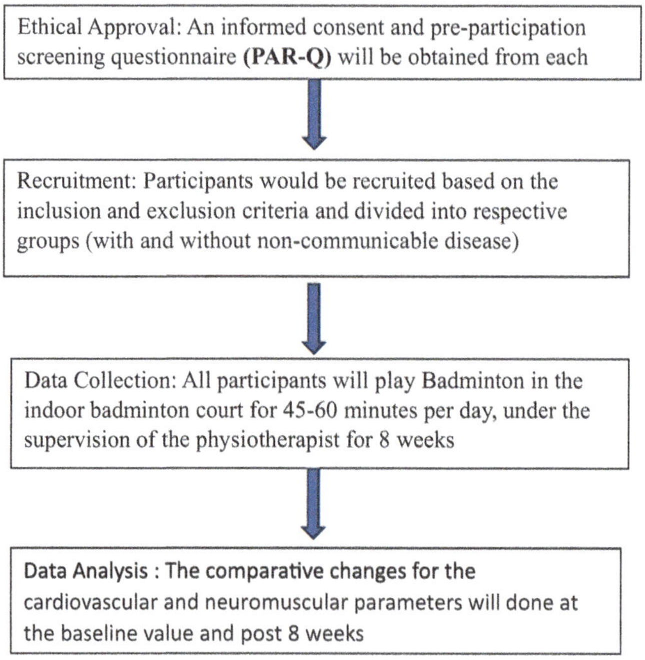

Fig. 8.1 Schematic representation of study procedure for documentation

8.1.4 *Writing Research Proposal Methodology for Physical Therapy Project: Worked Sample*

Title: Effect of Badminton Sports on Cardiovascular and Neuromuscular Parameters Among Older Adults with Noncommunicable Disease

Study Design: Observational, cross-sectional

Study Setting: Sport Complex, Gulf Medical University

Inclusion Criteria:

1. Age group: 55–70 years with three sub-age group divisions (55–60, 60–65, 65–70 years). Each sub-age group would consist of 14 participants making a total of 42 participants with noncommunicable group, and age- and gender-matched 42 participants without noncommunicable disease.
2. Both genders.
3. Participants without a history of noncommunicable disease and with noncommunicable disease (diabetes mellitus, hypertension, and obesity only). Stress is a composite disorder that would be assessed in the quality-of-life domain.

Exclusion Criteria:

Any joint disorders, cancer, neurologically unstable or prior physically active participants.

Study Procedure: The older adults would be divided into two groups, viz. (1) with noncommunicable diseases and (2) without noncommunicable diseases. Both groups would engage in badminton sports as per the specific inclusion and exclusion criteria. An informed consent shall be obtained from each participant after the ethical approval. Following this, participants would be recruited under purposive sampling from all seven emirates of the United Arab Emirates. All participants would be allowed to play badminton on the University's indoor court for 45–60 min/day. The protocol would be followed for 3 days a week at mild-to-moderate intensity under a supervised coach and physiotherapist for 2-month duration. The baseline physical activity level is assessed using the IPAQ questionnaire. The comparative changes in the cardiovascular and neuromuscular parameters shall be done at the value and post 2 months.

Study Outcome Variables and Measures:

The outcome measures would focus on physiological, biomechanical, and psychosocial parameters targeting the cardiovascular and neuromuscular functions.

(A) Noncommunicable disease parameters

- Blood sugar profile and HbA1c for diabetes mellitus
- Blood pressure values and lipid profile for hypertension
- Body mass index and hip waist circumference for obesity

(A) Cardiovascular Parameters

- VO_2 max analysis

(B) Musculoskeletal Parameters

- Muscle strength: tested using dynamometer and Oxford grading
- Muscle length for lower limb: clinical examination
- Agility: clinical test
- Lower limb joint power: force plates, motion analysis system
- Muscle peak force for quadriceps and hamstring: isokinetic device
- Trunk muscle balance: postural bench
- Muscle recruitment pattern: wireless electromyography

(C) Neuromuscular Parameters

- Proprioception
- Balance and coordination
- Reaction and response time
- Hand-eye coordination

(D) Quality of Life

The main study outcome would be to draw an interest in badminton sports among the older age groups. The study findings could allow coaches to identify the weak components of sports skills in the older age group and design their training accordingly. The BWF could expand its projects and training centers based on the preliminary findings of the research.

Research Timeline:

1st to 2nd Month: Ethical clearance
3rd to 12th Month: Participant recruitment and data collection
13th to 18th Month: Follow-up and data analysis
18th to 24th Month: Publication and presentation of findings

8.1.5 Summary

A well-developed research proposal would lay the path for accurate and current research output. The research proposal has major sections including an introduction, review of literature, and methodology, whereas the results, discussion, and conclusion are added after completion of data collection and data analysis.

References

Cole A, Gill TK, Shanahan EM, Phillips P, Taylor AW, Hill CL. Is diabetes associated with shoulder pain or stiffness? Results from a population based study. The Journal of Rheumatology. 2009 Feb 1;36(2):371–7.

Hunter SK, Pereira HM, Keenan KG. The aging neuromuscular system and motor performance. Journal of applied physiology. 2016 Oct 26.

Lawton E, Brymer E, Clough P, Denovan A. The relationship between the physical activity environment, nature relatedness, anxiety, and the psychological well-being benefits of regular exercisers. Frontiers in psychology. 2017 Jun 26;8:1058.

Wilkinson DJ, Piasecki M, Atherton PJ. The age-related loss of skeletal muscle mass and function: Measurement and physiology of muscle fibre atrophy and muscle fibre loss in humans. Ageing research reviews. 2018 Nov 1;47:123-32.

Chapter 9
Conducting Research: Scientific Methodological Rigor in Data Collection

9.1 Background

Conducting research with scientific methodological rigor is essential to ensure that the study produces reliable and valid results. Data collection is a crucial phase of the research process, and careful planning and execution are necessary to gather high-quality data. Although all components of research methodology should follow scientific rigor, we shall learn the salient point for conducting research with a rigorous methodology focused on the data collection procedure in this chapter. The following points should be addressed well to ensure that data collection for a given research has followed standard and rigorous procedures.

9.1.1 Standardization

The process of standardization is essential to ensure that the data collected is accurate and has no variability. In simple words, standardization means that there is high consistency in the collection of data from each participant and no difference should be observed in the procedure.

Example 9.1
A physical therapist wants to assess the knee joint force during squat jumps in females. The researcher will ensure that the procedure of the jump, environmental condition, instructions for the task, outfits, etc. which form the part of procedural technique should be the same for all participants during data collection. For instance, the researcher cannot conduct the jump test for one participant in shoes and another barefoot as it would lead to compromised methodological rigor and wrong data collection.

A. Hazari, *Research Methodology for Allied Health Professionals*,
https://doi.org/10.1007/978-981-99-8925-6_9

Example 9.2
A medical lab professional wants to determine the blood sugar level of patients undergoing angioplasty. It would be a wrong data collection procedure if the sugar levels were tested at different times for different participants. The researcher cannot collect the sample in the morning for one person and afternoon for another since there would be variations in the blood sugar level due to diurnal variation. Therefore, the researcher must follow a standard time, standard food, and standards of collecting the sample, which is equally applicable to all participants.

9.1.2 Instrumentation

To ensure that the data collection procedure is accurate and valid, the instruments or outcome measures used in the study should be well defined and selected with higher reliability and validity. To yield the best results in research, the ***gold standard*** tool/instruments or outcome measures should be used. In research, the gold standard tools have already been proposed for multiple outcome variables, which are commonly used for clinical research in allied health professions. For example, to determine the strength of muscle in physical therapy practice, an isokinetic device is the gold standard. However, it is possible that the researcher may not have the given facility or instrument at their prime study setting and therefore alternative tools could be used. Like instead of the isokinetic device, manual muscle testing (MMT) is often used in clinical practice. It should be noted that MMT may fail to produce the scientific rigor for data collection at master's and Ph.D. level research work. Thus, researchers must try to opt for the gold standard instruments for his/her study.

9.1.3 Questionnaire for Data Collection

For qualitative studies, research questionnaires are often used for data collection. A "questionnaire" is a tool for collecting information to describe, compare, or explain an event or situation, as well as knowledge, attitudes, behaviors, and/or sociodemographic characteristics on a particular target group. In common research practice, it could be used in three ways, viz. (1) self-administered (a questionnaire to be given to participants via email, personal contacts, advertisement, etc., and participants fill in the data as instructed), (2) in person which is through one-to-one contact, and (3) telephonic interviews.

These questionnaires enable the researcher to collect data that could be coded further to quantify and interpret the results. There are multiple questionnaires developed for various outcome variables to be tested in allied health professionals. These questionnaires are easily available and validated against gold standards. However, researchers may find difficulty at times in the application of already published questionnaires, and the need to design their questionnaire may arise. Designing research questionnaires is a researcher's freedom, but it should have good validity and reliability as a requirement for any outcome measures. Failure to use or design a good research questionnaire may affect the accuracy of the data collected. Examples of research questionnaires used in physical therapy practice include quality-of-life tools, diabetes neuropathy screening tools, pain questionnaires, etc.

9.1.4 Developing Research Questionnaire

As discussed above, researchers may feel a need to design and develop their questionnaire for their research study. The questions or items used in the questionnaire should directly relate to the theme of the proposed research and give information about its objectives. Also, the response should target the desired outcome variables. For example, if a study wants to understand the pain level of a construction worker through a self-administered questionnaire, it should not ask about their quality of life until and unless that falls under the objectives of the study. Therefore, the items used in the questionnaire should be as limited and focused as possible. The questions used in the research questionnaire are basically of two types: open-ended and closed-ended.

9.1.4.1 Open-ended

The open-ended questions allow the participants to be more expressive as they have the freedom to provide the information without restriction, but it is very difficult to analyze them for research purposes. For example, a medical lab researcher asks an open-ended question to his diabetes mellitus subjects as quoted.

"How do you feel in the morning when you get up"? The participants have the freedom to answer multiple expressions such as lazy, happy, irritated, and sleepy. Considering that the sample size for the research study is 100 and 80 different responses are given, the researcher will have to face serious difficulties in analysis. In such cases, the qualitative data could be coded for quantitative analysis, for example, use of the Likert scale. The researcher can code common responses and produce the data. An example of a workout can be seen in the next chapter.

9.1.4.2 Closed-ended

To avoid such issues related to difficulty in analysis, closed-ended questions are maximally used in research practices. The same question can be given to participants "Do you feel weak when you get up?" Yes/No. The participant would have an option to choose, making it a closed-ended response for easy understanding, coding, analyzing, and reporting.

9.1.4.3 Categories of Closed-Ended Questions

As discussed, researchers should look to use the closed-ended questionnaire for easy analysis and interpretation in research. The following three categories of questions can be targeted to develop research questionnaires/tools.

(a) Nominal

- What is your gender?
  - Female
  - Male
- What is your marital status?
  - Single
  - Married
  - Widowed

(b) Ordinal

- What is your age?
  - <15
  - 16–20
  - 21–30
  - 31–49
  - 50 and over
- What is the level of you pain?
  - Mild
  - Moderate
  - Severe

(c) Numerical

- Rate your pain on a scale of 1–10 (1 least pain and 10 maximum pain).
- How many cigarettes do you smoke in a day?
- What is the frequency of urination per hour for a diabetic patient?

9.1.5 Validating Research Questionnaire

The scientific rigor for data collection through research questionnaires majorly depends upon its validity. After designing a research questionnaire, it is important to validate it for use in research purposes. Validating a research questionnaire is a critical step to ensure that the questions developed are clear, relevant, and reliable. Researchers are advised to follow the given steps to validate their research questionnaire before administration to participants.

9.1.5.1 Pilot Testing

It involves conducting a test with a small sample of individuals who closely represent the target population. This will help to identify any issues with the questionnaire's clarity, wording, or instructions. It would be good to choose a diverse group of participants to get varied perspectives.

9.1.5.2 Face Validity

This consists of reviewing the questionnaire by own self (researcher) to ensure that the questions appear to measure what they are intended to measure. Check for any ambiguities, unclear terms, or irrelevant questions.

9.1.5.3 Expert Review

Experts in the field of allied health sciences (in context to this book) or any field could be used to review the questionnaire who can provide valuable feedback on the relevance, clarity, and appropriateness of the questions. They can also help ensure that the questionnaire aligns with established theories and concepts to meet the research requirements.

9.1.5.4 Content Validity

This involves assessing the contents of the questionnaire by checking whether the questions cover all the relevant aspects of the topic being researched. It is important to ensure that there is a good balance of questions that address different dimensions of your research.

9.1.5.5 Construct Validity

This refers to whether the questionnaire accurately measures the underlying constructs or concepts we are interested in. To assess construct validity, researchers can use established scales or compare the developed questionnaire to similar instruments that have already been validated. For example, if a physical therapist wants to develop a quality-of-life questionnaire for construction workers, he/she can validate the questionnaire again, WHO QoL or SF-36.

9.1.5.6 Criterion Validity

If you have access to external criteria, you can assess the extent to which your questionnaire's results correlate with these criteria. This can provide evidence of criterion validity. It may not be applicable for major research in allied health professionals.

9.1.5.7 Reliability

As defined before, it refers to the consistency and stability of your questionnaire's results. Researchers can assess reliability through methods like test-retest reliability (administering the questionnaire twice to the same group with some time in between) or internal consistency (using techniques like Cronbach's alpha for Likert-type scales).

9.1.6 Summary

Scientific rigor is important for data collection in research methodology. The data collection procedure must follow the process of standardization. It is important to use the gold standard instruments for data accuracy. When there is a need to design research questionnaires, they should be validated and developed with a focus on meeting the research objectives.

Chapter 10
Data Analysis: Descriptive and Analytical Statistics

10.1 Background

The analysis of the raw data is very important to make meaningful interpretations while also testing the research hypothesis. The process of data analysis in research involves data redundancy, integration, filtration, and statistical processing. Each step has been explained below. All researchers need to perform data analysis with accuracy after the collection of data. The raw data often does not provide meaningful results and thus needs to be processed for better understanding and provide a scientific conclusion to the research hypothesis by either accepting or rejecting it.

10.1.1 Data Redundancy

In research, data redundancy refers to the duplication of data within a dataset or across multiple datasets. Redundancy can occur for various reasons, including data entry errors, data integration processes, and data backup strategies. Therefore, managing data redundancy is essential to ensure data accuracy, consistency, and efficiency. Once the raw data has been obtained, the important variables are extracted as per the research objective.

10.1.2 Data Integration and Filtration

After the raw data is extracted, the data needs to be integrated as primary and secondary variables following which some of the data may require to go through a process of filtering. For example, a physical therapist conducted a 3D motion

A. Hazari, *Research Methodology for Allied Health Professionals*,
https://doi.org/10.1007/978-981-99-8925-6_10

analysis of cerebral palsy gait, and his objective was to determine the ankle joint range of motion at the heel strike and toe-off phase of the gait cycle. The raw data has been integrated into the Excel sheet, which provides the coordinates of the lower limb joint. The research would need to extract the information and filter it for further analysis of joint angles into degrees or radians. In simple words, the process of data filtration is refining the data to shape it into presentable results such as tables, pie charts, and histograms.

10.1.3 Data Normalization

At times, the raw data would need to be normalized to a given standard for its applicability to generalize the findings in context to the given research. The process of normalization becomes a must when there is too much variability in the raw data, and it would be difficult to compare and interpret the findings of the results. Also known as data scaling, it is a crucial step in data preprocessing for research and analysis. It involves transforming data into a common scale or range to ensure that different features or variables have equal influence on the analysis, especially when using algorithms that are sensitive to the magnitude of data. Normalization can also improve the convergence of machine learning algorithms and make the data more interpretable. Let us understand this with the following example.

Example: An anesthesia technician is researching determining the optimal dose of sedation in a diabetic patient through a general anesthesia drug.

Now the dose of the drug needs to be decided depending on certain factors of the individual such as age, body weight, and hyperglycemic state. The researcher has collected a dataset with the following information for a sample:

Age ranging from 30 to 70 years

Body weight ranging from 58 to 104 kg

The hyperglycemic state recorded by random blood sugar level (RBS) ranging from 189 to 294 mg/dL

Before performing any analysis or building a predictive model, we need to normalize the data because the scales of these variables are different. In most of the health research, we can use the following formulas for normalization:

10.1.3.1 Min-Max Scaling (Normalization)

In min-max scaling, you transform the data to a specific range, typically between 0 (min) and 1 (max). The formula for min-max scaling is:

$$X_{normalized} = \left(X - X_{min}\right) / \left(X_{max} - X_{min}\right)$$

10.1.3.2 Z-Score Standardization

Z-score standardization transforms the data to have a mean of 0 and a standard deviation of 1. The formula for z-score standardization is:

$$X\,\text{standardized} = \left(X - \mu\right) / \sigma$$

where

X = actual observation
μ = mean of the variable
σ = standard deviation of the variable

After normalizing the data, all the features will be on the same scale, making it easier to compare and analyze them. This ensures that, for example, the younger person with lesser body weight and less RBS contributes equally to the model for dose prediction as an older person with higher body weight and higher RBS value would contribute to determining the dose.

10.1.4 Statistical Analysis: Descriptive and Analytical

After the raw data has been integrated, filtered, and scaled where applicable, the data needs to be analyzed for statistical inferences. The data can be statistically analyzed and categorized into descriptive or analytical as explained with examples below:

10.1.4.1 Descriptive Statistics

Descriptive statistics are a set of methods and techniques used to summarize and directly describe the main findings of a dataset or a sample. They provide a way to understand and interpret data by presenting key information about its central tendency, variability, and distribution. Descriptive statistics are often the first step in data analysis and are essential for gaining insights into a dataset before more advanced statistical methods are applied. Here are some of the most common descriptive statistics:

Measures of Central Tendency

Mean: The arithmetic average of all values in the dataset. It is calculated by summing up all values and dividing them by the number of values.

Example: A researcher has 100 samples in a study, and he wants to represent the demographic data of all participants which include age, height, and weight. He/she would conduct a descriptive statistic to obtain the mean and standard deviation of the desired demographic variables.

Median: The middle value in a dataset when it is ordered from smallest to largest. It is less sensitive to extreme values (outliers) compared to the mean.

Example: A researcher wants to report the average IQ level of autistic children in his study. Standardization in the data collection has been maintained as participants belong to the same class, ethnicity, geographical area, and similar socioeconomic characteristics. He would not use mean here as mean would be affected by the extreme values, and it would not represent the average IQ level correctly for the given sample. Here, median should be used instead of the mean.

Mode: The value that occurs most frequently in the dataset. A dataset can have no mode, one mode (unimodal), or multiple modes (multimodal).

Example: A researcher wants to report the highest scores by all toppers from standard 1 to standard 12 in English subject. Here, the mode would be suitable to represent the proposed research objective.

Measures of Variability or Dispersion

Range: The difference between the maximum and minimum values in the dataset. It provides a simple measure of the spread of data.

Example: A researcher wants to determine the range of blood sugar levels for his sample population in the research. He would note the lowest value and the highest value, and the difference would be expressed as the range.

Variance: A measure of how much the data points deviate from the mean. It is the average of the squared differences between each data point and the mean.

Example: A researcher wants to identify the change in the blood sugar level following 8 weeks of aerobic training. Here, the variance would be calculated as the deviation from the mean.

Standard Deviation: The square root of the variance. It measures the average distance between each data point and the mean, providing a more interpretable measure of dispersion.

Measures of Shape and Distribution

Skewness: A measure of the asymmetry of the data distribution. The researchers report their dataset within the 95% confidence interval (CI) ranging from $-2\ \sigma$ to $+2\ \sigma$ (standard deviation) on the normal distribution curve (Fig. 10.1). Positive skewness indicates a longer tail on the right side (Fig. 10.2), while negative skewness indicates a longer tail on the left side of a normal distribution curve as shown in Fig. 10.3. If the observations are more towards the positive side of the mean, it is positively skewed and vice versa.

Kurtosis: A measure of the "tailedness" of the data distribution. It indicates whether the data has heavy tails or is more peaked compared to a normal

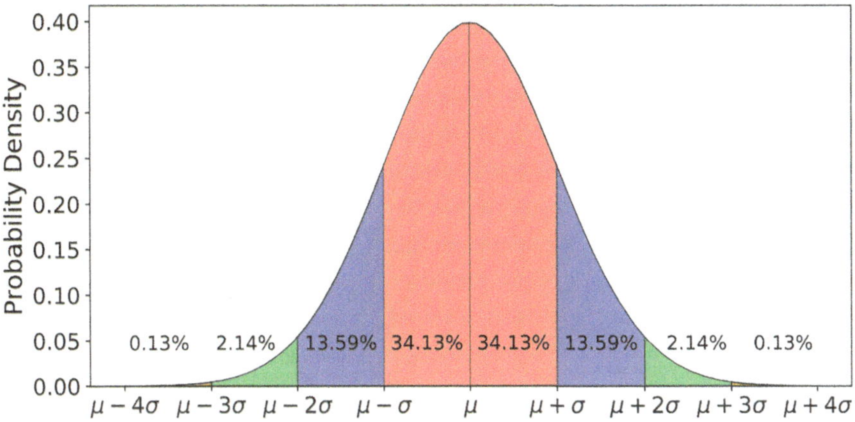

Fig. 10.1 Normal distribution curve of the data sample

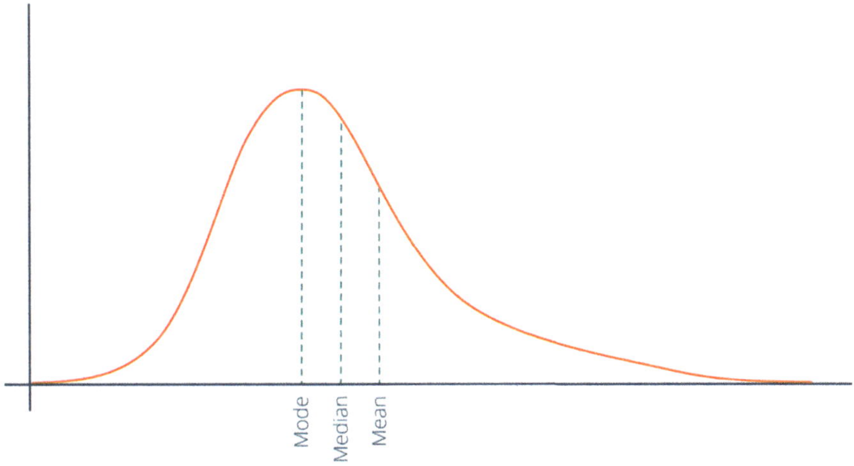

Fig. 10.2 Positively skewed dataset on a normal distribution curve. Note: mean > median > mode

distribution. Data could be represented as ***"leptokurtic"*** (high peaked), "***mesokurtic"*** (medium peaked), and "***platykurtic***" (least peaked or flat).

Example: A researcher wants to compare the highest scores of toppers in standards 5, 10, and 12 for science subjects (out of 100). His findings report a mean score of 96 in standard 5, 84 in standard 10, and 71 in standard 12. The data can be represented on a normal distribution curve for kurtosis.

Percentiles: Values that divide the dataset into 100 equal parts. The 25th, 50th (median), and 75th percentiles are commonly used to describe data in allied health streams.

Example: A physical therapist wants to determine the normative value of biceps strength among university female students. The researcher would need to first take

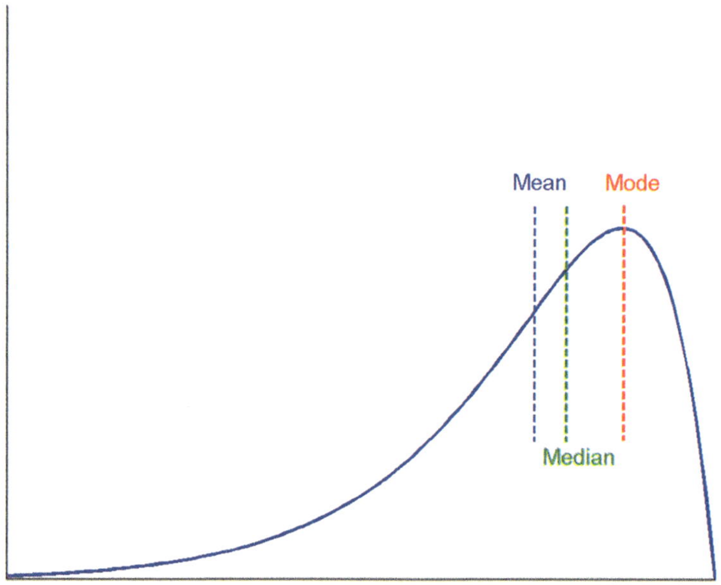

Fig. 10.3 Negatively skewed dataset on a normal distribution curve. Note: mean < median < mode

the mean peak strength and report the data for individuals as a percentile for normative values.

Frequency Distribution: A table or graph that shows how often each value or range of values occurs in the dataset. Histograms and bar charts are often used to visualize frequency distributions.

Example: A researcher wants to determine the frequency of smoking and drinking among construction workers in each industry.

Percentage: Represented as values from 0% to 100% and most used for survey studies such as reporting prevalence rates.

10.1.4.2 Analytical Statistics

Also known as "inferential statistics," which involves using data from a sample to make inferences or draw conclusions about a larger population. Unlike descriptive statistics, which summarize and describe data, analytical statistics focus on testing hypotheses, making predictions, and generalizing findings for a given research study. The inferential stats are often used by researchers and are categorized into **"parametric tests"** and **"nonparametric tests"** as discussed below.

Parametric Tests

The parametric tests are used to test a research hypothesis when the data collected by the researcher shows normal distribution. In simple words, data is not skewed and falls within the 95% confidence interval as demonstrated in Fig. 10.1, suggesting that all observations are evenly distributed. Commonly used parametric tests include t-tests, chi-squared tests, regression, and analysis of variance (ANOVA). In statistics, there are important assumptions to use the parametric tests as listed below:

- Normality: Data in each group should be normally distributed (the steps of conducting a normal distribution test have been given in the next section).
- Independence: Data in each group should be sampled randomly and independently.
- No outliers: No extreme outliers in the data.
- Equal variance: Data in each group should have approximately equal variance.

Nonparametric Tests

These tests are used when data do not meet the assumptions of parametric tests (e.g., normal distribution). The most common examples include the Wilcoxon rank-sum test and the Kruskal-Wallis test.

Note: The analytical tests are conducted using advanced software and statistical tools. Researchers can use any of the software packages depending on the availability, ease of use, and expertise.

10.1.5 Statistical Analysis Software

Analytical statistics often involves the use of statistical software packages like R, Python (with libraries like NumPy, SciPy, and scikit-learn), SAS, SPSS, and others to perform data analysis and hypothesis testing. Within the scope of this book, we shall learn how to use the SPSS (Statistical Package for Social Sciences) as it is preferred by most of the allied health professionals to serve their research purposes. It would be advisable to refer to other statistics books to learn other softwares.

10.1.6 SPSS

It is a useful data analysis package that allows complex and high volumes of data analysis in a quick time. This software is used by many allied health researchers and provides extremely thorough and well-presented analyses. Let us learn how to use SPSS in a stepwise manner with worked-out examples. For demonstration, the available licensed version has been used here. Researchers are free to use the latest or any version.

10.1.6.1 Defining Variables and Data Entry in SPSS

The first step in using SPSS is to define your variables (both dependent and independent) as instructed here.

Step 1: Install the SPSS package on your systems (latest version or licensed version).

Step 2: Launch SPSS, and you will be faced with the following windows (Fig. 10.4).

Step 3: Defining variable names: To define variables, click on the "Variable View" tab—the layout of the window will change (Fig. 10.5); in this view, each variable has a row to itself—variable 1 in row 1, variable 2 in row 2, and so on. You will see that there are several column headers, such as Name, Type, and Width. These are important characteristics that you can change for each variable.

Step 4: Data entry: After the variables have been defined, click the "Data View" tab for data entry. A new window would open as shown in Fig. 10.6. SPSS is very specific about how the data should be laid out. It must be presented in the correct format if statistical tests are to be carried out correctly:

- Each subject has **only one row** (numbered 1, 2, 3, etc.). Therefore, data entry should be in the row as per the defined variables. For example, if a researcher has defined a variable as height, then for each participant, data for height would be entered in separate rows.
- The column headers (all initially showing "var") will contain the variable(s) for the subject as defined by the researcher.

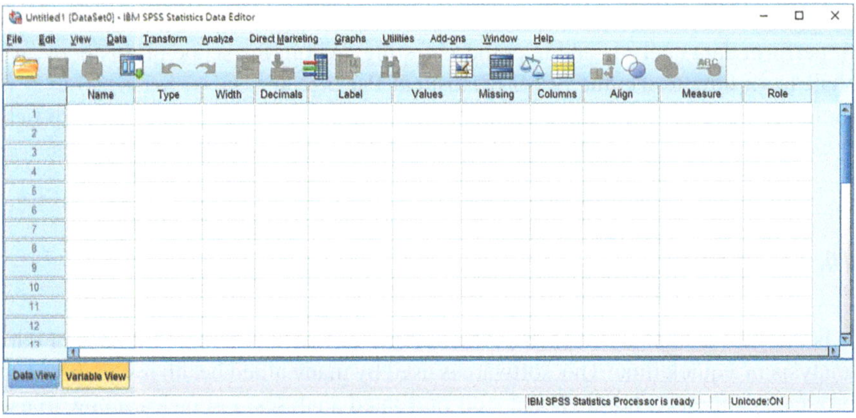

Fig. 10.4 SPSS layout for data and variable entry

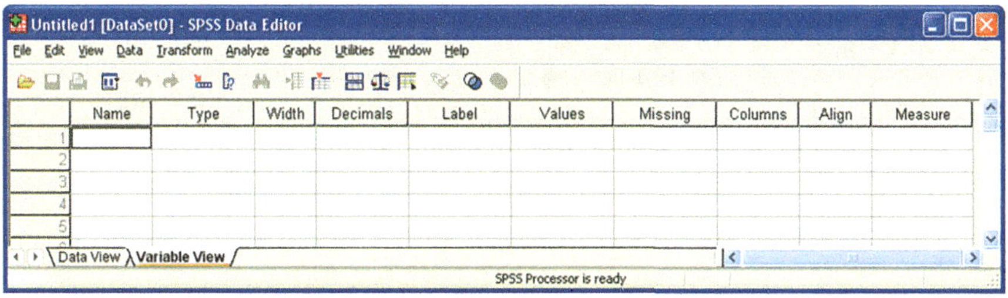

Fig. 10.5 Variable view for defining variables

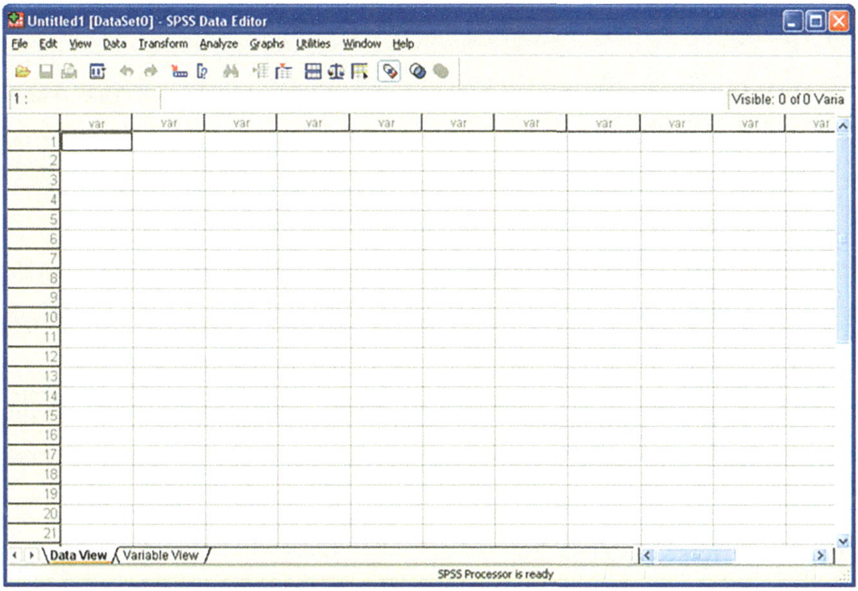

Fig. 10.6 Data view for data entry

Data Entry: Worked Example 1

In Example 1 below (where we will only be setting up a data file at this stage), a group of six subjects are tested to see how many mental arithmetic questions they can answer correctly in a set time, in two different environmental conditions: Quiet music and Loud music. Since the same subject is being tested more than once (repeated measures within the subject study), we will need to build the data table so that the values are entered in the same row. Our data then is a pair of values for each subject: a reading for under the "Quiet" condition and another for the "Loud" condition. Therefore, Quiet and Loud are our variables in this example. We would start with the Variable View. In row 1, in the column marked Name, type Quiet, our first variable, and then press the down arrow key. The active cell will now change to the second row name field, where you should enter Loud (Fig. 10.7).

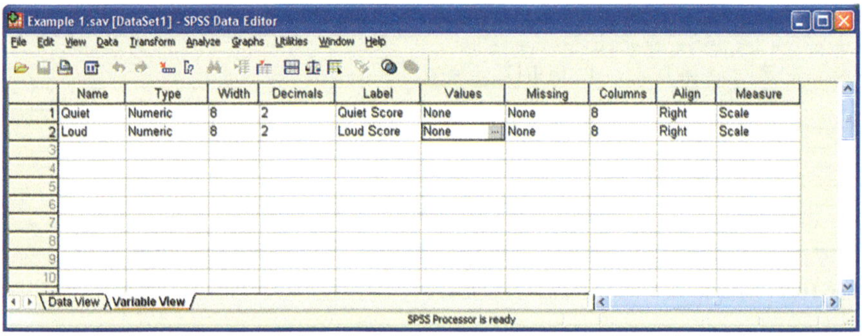

Fig. 10.7 Variable setup

Table 10.1 Dataset for entry in SPSS (worked example 1)

Quiet	Loud
14	12
10	11
9	8
16	15
12	13
15	14

Now, with our variables defined, click back on **Data View** so that we can enter the below sample data from the data collection sheet (Table 10.1). After the data entry, our window should appear as shown in Fig. 10.8.

Data Entry: Worked Example 2

In this example, the researcher decided to recruit 12 participants and assign them to one of the conditions (Quiet or Loud) so that each subject is only tested once, unlike the first example where the participants were assigned to both. We have two groups of subjects: six for tests under "Quiet" conditions and six for tests under "Loud."

Since we want to look at groups now, we must tell SPSS that we are dealing with a variable that is composed of two groups—Quiet and Loud. So, our variables this time are group and sums for each participant. As before, enter the names of the variables, and our window should appear as shown in Fig. 10.9.

However, the variable "group" has two possible values, which we need to encode. Let us represent the Quiet group with a number 1 and the Loud group with a number 2. That is, whenever we enter 1 in the data table, we wish SPSS to identify this as a member of the Quiet group and 2 to mean from the Loud group. To do this, click on the Values column in the group variable—and then once on the three-dot ellipses which will appear on the right-hand side of the cell, in a grey box. A "Values Labels" dialogue box should appear as shown in Fig. 10.10.

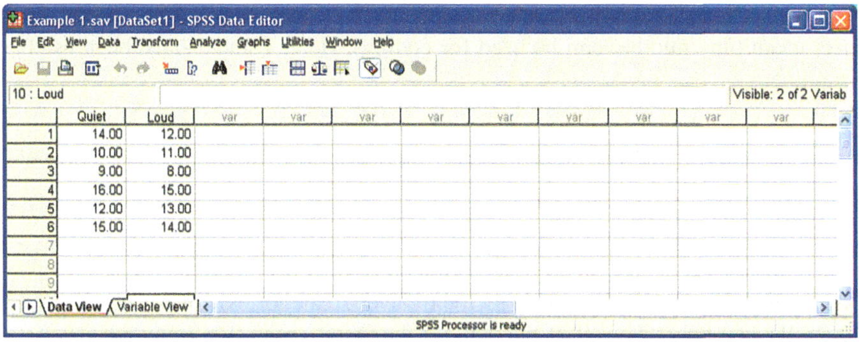

Fig. 10.8 Data entry for worked example 1

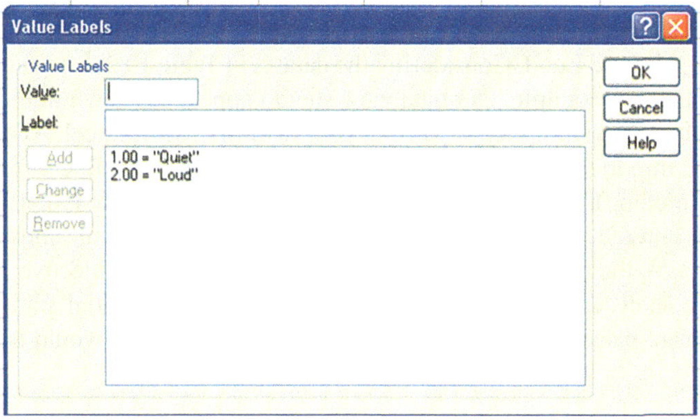

Fig. 10.10 Coding for variables defined as "group" in the worked example 2

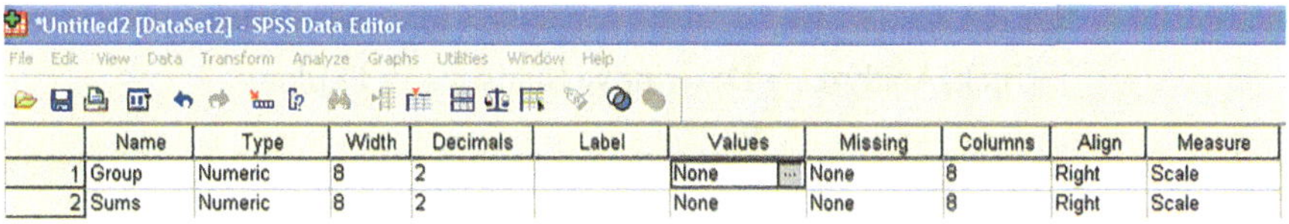

Fig. 10.9 Defining variables for worked example 2

Now we need to assign a number to the "Value" box to tell SPSS what the numbers mean (any number can be used for coding). Here, 1 and 2 have been used as example.

- In the Value box, type 1.
- In the Value Label box, type "Quiet" and then click "add" (the instruction will drop down into the box below).
- Repeat this, so that 2 = Loud.

We have now encoded our groups Quiet and Loud as numbers 1 and 2, respectively (Fig. 10.10). We can code as many levels (categories) for a variable as we wish. We can now enter all of the data for the Quiet group first (remember that we have six subjects in each group), so in the first six rows (a row per subject), type the number 1 in the Group column, to show that it is a Quiet condition subject and in rows 7–12, enter number 2 in the Group column for the Loud condition subjects. If we click on the symbol arrowed, the numbers 1 and 2 will be shown in their decoded form, i.e., Quiet and Loud. Considering the dataset in Table 10.2, let us complete the data entry for this example. Our data view should appear as shown in Fig. 10.11.

Note: There is a similarity of SPSS layout with Microsoft Excel. Also, although data can be imported from other software packages, including Excel (using a "cut and paste" method), it is very important not to consider SPSS like Excel, in terms of how data is entered and analyzed; the cell-based layout is where the similarity ends!

We can save the file for further analysis as per the research objective. In the next section, we shall learn how to conduct descriptive and inferential statistics in the SPSS software package. The same example as discussed above would be referred.

10.1.7 Conducting Descriptive Statistics in SPSS

It is very simple and quick to analyze our research data using the descriptive analysis method in the SPSS. Once the dataset is ready, use the following steps to run the descriptive analyses:

$$\text{Click, Analyze} \rightarrow \text{Descriptive Statistics} \rightarrow \text{Explore}$$

Table 10.2 Dataset for entry in SPSS (worked example 2)

Quiet	Loud
13	14
15	9
16	12
7	10
10	15
12	9

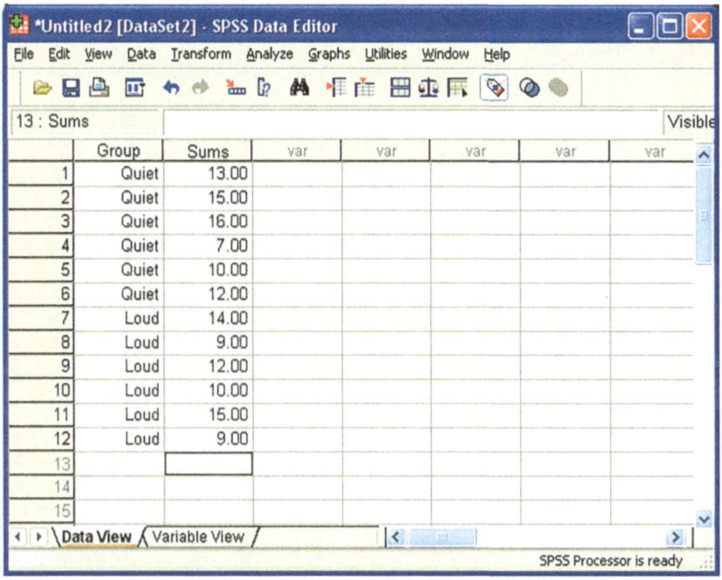

Fig. 10.11 Data entry for worked example 2

A small command window will now open. Click once on the name of the columns (variables to be analyzed) you have, and then click the little arrow tab beside the Dependent List box. Do this for each variable in turn, and they will each in turn transfer across from the left-hand box into the Dependent List box. Once both columns are there, click Statistics under the Display section of the window and then click OK.

When SPSS performs a calculation or a test, it puts the results in a new window labeled Output as this is the first calculation you have done. The window will be labeled Output 1 and will contain the Explore output for the two data columns from example 1. Scroll down, and you will see you have the main descriptive statistics for each column, so for example you can now compare means and standard deviation across columns.

10.1.8 Conducting Inferential Statistics in SPSS

We will now learn to run inferential statistics through SPSS. The first step is to conduct the test for normality and then decide the appropriate parametric and nonparametric tests as shown in the diagram in Fig. 10.12. This flowchart may not include all statistical tests; however, it would be helpful to guide most of the researchers in the allied health stream.

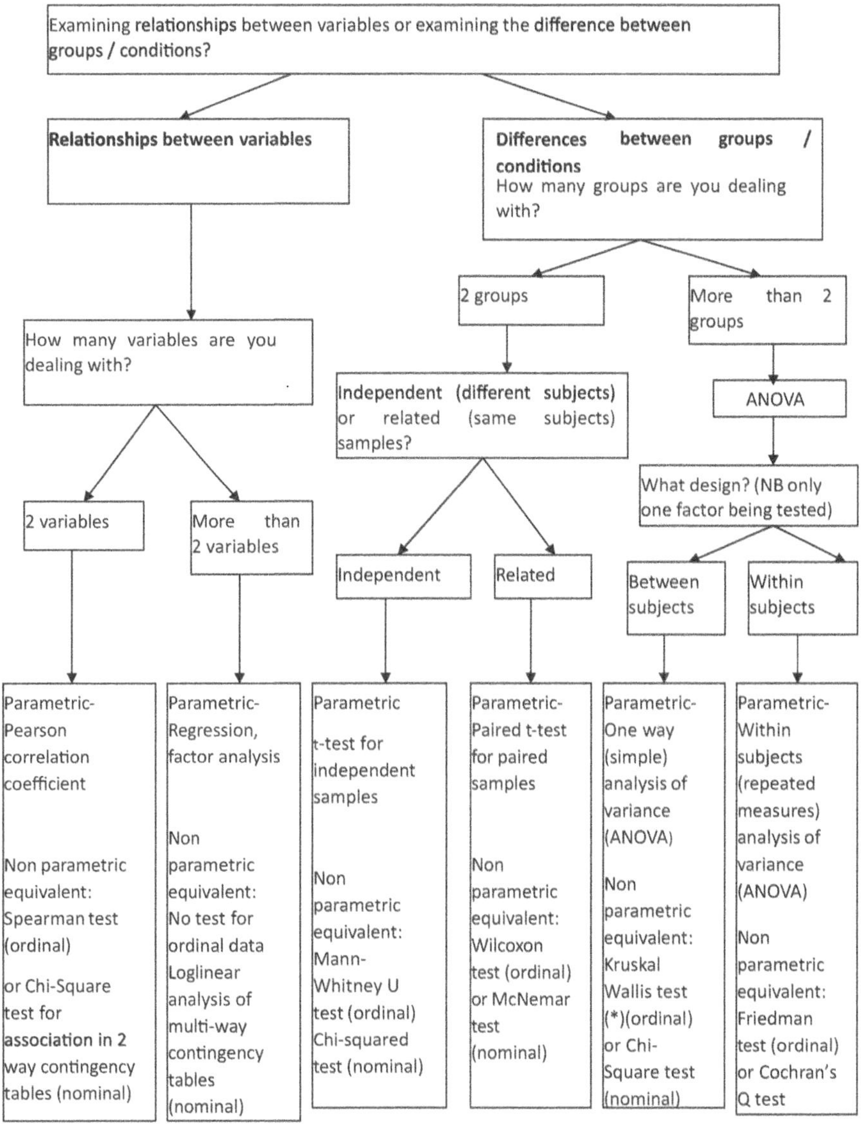

Fig. 10.12 Flow diagram for using correct inferential statistic tests

10.1.8.1 Test for Normal Distribution of Data

It is always important to test the data for normal distribution since the selection of parametric and nonparametric tests depends heavily on this assumption. The researcher can be confident that the data has achieved an important assumption for parametric testing. If the number of observations is less than 50 ($n < 50$), it would be suitable to use the Shapiro-Wilk test, whereas if the number is higher, the Kolmogorov-Smirnov test would be a better indicator for the test of normality.

How to Calculate a Test of Normality of Distribution Using SPSS

- Click Analyze—Descriptive Statistics—Explore
- Transfer the variable name of the data you want to look at into the Dependent List box.
- Check the Both mini button in the display box.
- Click the Plots button, select Normality plots with test, and then Continue.
- Click OK.

How to Interpret the SPSS Test of Normality of Distribution Output

Check the output table for the Tests of Normality table, which gives the significance of both the Kolmogorov-Smirnov (KS) and Shapiro-Wilk (SW) test statistics. For both tests (KS and SW), a value greater than 0.05 in the Sig. Column of the output table indicates that the data can be treated as normally distributed and parametric testing could be done. It is important to test each dataset for each variable for normality distribution.

10.1.8.2 Conduction and Interpretation of Independent T-Test

An independent t-test is commonly used to find out if there is a difference between two variables/subjects/samples. The test is used for an experimental design, which aims to compare two different groups of subjects being independent of each other. In simple words, it is most suitable for "between-group analysis."

Example 10.1
A physical therapist wants to compare the quadriceps strength between footballers and basketball players. It suggests that it is a between-group analysis, and since footballers and basketball players are different groups with different characteristics, an independent t-test should be used if the data is normally distributed. If data is not normally distributed, the nonparametric equivalent Mann-Whitney U test should be applied.

How to Compute an Independent T-Test Using SPSS

- Perform data entry in SPSS. Ensure that you have a column with a defined group and that you have no more than two groups represented in that column.
- Click Analyze—Compare means—Independent-samples T-test.

- Click on the dependent variable, and click the little arrow to place it in the Test Variable(s) box.
- Click on Group, and click the arrow to place it in the Grouping Variable(s) box (Define the group).
- Click continue, and then click OK.

How to Interpret and Report the SPSS Output of an Independent T-Test

The top table of the output provides details of the descriptive statistics. The bottom table shows the test statistics, which are divided into two lines based on whether there are equal variances between the different conditions. The key to whether equal variances can or cannot be assumed lies in the outcome of Levene's test for equality of variances, which is listed as part of the SPSS output. This is a test for the homogeneity of variance assumption of a valid t-test. Provided that the test is not significant ($p > 0.05$), the variances can be assumed to be homogeneous, and the equal variances line for the t-test can be used. In Levene's test, if $p > 0.5$, then the top line of the SPSS output is used. If $p < 0.5$, then the bottom line of the SPSS output is used. The test statistics table provides the difference between the two sample means as well as the standard deviation and standard error of the mean. The 95% confidence limit is also provided. Confidence limits are provided to help reinforce the results obtained in the t-test. The lower and upper levels of the confidence limits inform you of the boundaries that the mean differences of the variables must lie between for us to be 95% confident that the results are not due to chance or random error. The values that you are particularly interested in are the t value and the probability (p) value.

10.1.8.3 Conduction and Interpretation of Paired T-Test

The paired t-test or the dependent t-test is used when testing for significant differences between two samples/groups/observations, which are related. In simple words, it can be regarded as within-group analysis. For example, in Sect. 10.1.8.1, if the researcher wants to identify the quadriceps strength in the same participant while playing football and basketball, a paired t-test should be applied if the data is normally distributed. The nonparametric equivalent to this test is the Wilcoxon test.

How to Compute a Paired T-Test Using SPSS

- Enter the relevant data into the Data Editor. Unlike with an independent t-test, there are no groups to define. Ensure that the two sets of data are typed in separate columns and labeled differently.
- Click Analyze—Compare means—Paired-samples T-test.

- Click on the names of both variables, which moves them down into the Current Selections box, and then click the little arrow which moves them into the Paired Variables text box.
- Click OK.

How to Interpret and Report the SPSS Output of a Paired T-Test

Three tables are produced in the output. The first shows descriptive statistics, the second shows the Pearson correlation between the two sets of scores, and the last table shows the test statistics (paired t-test). This last table provides us with the difference between the two sample means as well as the standard deviation and standard error of the mean. The values of interest are the t value and the probability (p) value.

10.1.8.4 Conduction and Interpretation of Analysis of Variance (ANOVA)

ANOVA is a parametric test like a t-test, but it is applied when the difference in means for more than two groups needs to be analyzed. For most of the research in the allied health stream, (simple) ANOVA or one-way ANOVA and within-subjects (repeated measures) ANOVA are used. In the ANOVA, a factor refers to a set of related conditions and is comparable to the terms independent variable and dependent variable used in a t-test.

In the simple ANOVA, the factors are between subjects and each subject is tested only once under one condition (i.e., at one level) of the factor. In repeated measures, ANOVA subjects are tested more than once under all the different conditions (levels) making up the factor and are said to have repeated measures on the factor. Considering the example given in Sects. 10.1.8.1 and 10.1.8.2, if the researchers want to compare the quadriceps strength of footballers and basketball players while jumping and running, then repeated measures ANOVA should be applied as here the comparison is at two levels. An example of one-way ANOVA would be comparing mean scores of the biomechanics term examination between three different groups of physiotherapy students including ten 1st-year students, ten 2nd-year students, and ten 3rd-year students. The nonparametric equivalents (for ordinal data) to the simple ANOVA and repeated measures ANOVA are the Kruskal-Wallis test and Friedman test, respectively.

How to Compute a Simple ANOVA Using SPSS

- Click Analyze—Compare means—One-way ANOVA.
- Define your dependent (outcome) variable, and place it in the Dependent List box.
- Select the Factor name (the name of the column where all your subjects have been listed with the various conditions defined), and move it into the Factor box.

- Click on Post Hoc—Scheffé—Continue.
- Click on Options—Descriptives—Homogeneity of Variance.

How to Interpret and Report the SPSS Output of a Simple ANOVA

The top sub-table provides descriptive statistics, with the means indicating where statistically significant differences between the means may lie. The second sub-table shows Levene's test for homogeneity of variance—a significant value ($p > 0.05$) in this test indicates that homogeneity can be assumed. The main ANOVA table appears next showing the F score and the exact significance value (p). A p-value of less than 0.05 indicates that there is a statistically significant difference between the means of the different conditions. The post hoc table can then inform you of where those differences lie and their level of significance.

How to Compute a Repeated Measures ANOVA Using SPSS

- Analyze—General Linear Model—Repeated Measures
- In the Within Subject Factor Name box, type the factor name (the name of the column where all your subjects have been listed with the various conditions defined).
- Type the number of levels of the within-subject variable in the Number of Levels box (i.e., the number of different conditions you are testing between), and click Add.
- Select Define, and click on the relevant variable names that define your conditions and move them to the Within-Subjects Variables box.
- Select Options, and in the Display box, click Descriptive Statistics.
- Click on Continue—OK.

How to Interpret and Report the SPSS Output of a Repeated Measures ANOVA

The first table lists the different conditions being tested with the second table providing descriptive data. The means listed in this table can indicate where statistically significant differences between the means may lie. The next table is Mauchly's test for sphericity—if the outcome of this test is not significant ($p > 0.05$), then sphericity can be assumed, and the appropriate row of the ANOVA table is followed. If $p < 0.05$, then a more conservative test is employed, and the Greenhouse-Geisser row should be followed in the ANOVA table. In the tests of the within-subjects effects ANOVA table, the F score and p-value are provided which is assumed to be significant if $p < 0.05$.

10.1.8.5 Correlation and Regression: Exploring the Relationship Between Two Variables

At times, a researcher is interested in finding out whether two variables are associated or linked. Correlation is the method of analysis used when studying the possible association between two continuous variables and the direction and strength of the association (strong or weak association, negative or positive association). Let us learn how to run a correlation stat in SPSS.

How to Compute a Pearson Correlation Using SPSS

- Enter the relevant data.
- Click Analyze—Correlate—Bivariate (two variables).
- Double-click on each variable in turn, and move them to the variable(s) box.
- Click OK.

How to Produce a Scatterplot Using SPSS

- Click Graph—Scatter.
- Select Simple as the default mode, and click on Define.
- Move the two variables into the box, and click OK.

To add a line of best-fit

- Double-click on the graph to bring up the SPSS Chart Editor.
- Click Chart—Options—Fit Line—Total—OK.

How to Interpret and Report the SPSS Output for a Pearson Correlation

There are two variables, so a 2 × 2 correlation matrix is formed. The correlation between the two variables is quoted as the r value in the table. The level of significance is set as $p < 0.05$.

10.1.8.6 Regression Analysis

Like correlation, regression looks at the association or relationship between two or more variables. It can help to establish a cause-and-effect relationship between the dependent and independent variables. Linear or multiple regression analyses can be used.

How to Compute a Regression Line Using SPSS

- Enter the relevant data.
- Click Analyze—regression—linear.
- Click on the dependent variable (the variable being predicted), and move it to the dependent variable box.
- Click on the independent variable, move it to the independent variable box, and click OK.

10.1.8.7 Chi-Square Analysis

This test is used when you wish to explore the relationship between two categorical variables: for example, finding a relationship for alcoholic behavior (yes or no) between male and female.

How to Compute a Chi-Square Using SPSS

- Click Analyze, then click on Descriptive Statistics, and then on Cross tabs.
- Click on one of your variables (e.g., Gender) to be your row variable, and click on the arrow to move it into the box marked Rows.
- Click on the other variable to be your column variable (e.g., Alcoholic), and click on the arrow to move it into the box marked Column.
- Click on the Statistics button. Choose Chi-square. Click on Continue.
- Click on the cells button.
- In the Counts box, click on the Observed and Expected boxes.
- In the Percentage section, click on the Row, Column, and Total boxes.
- Click on Continue and then OK.

10.1.9 Summary

Statistical analysis is one of the most essential components of research methodology, which is all about the processing of raw data for meaningful interpretation. Significant statistical data can be confidently generalized to the entire population as measured within the 95% confidence interval. The selection of the correct statistical method is the key to research methodology.

Chapter 11
Manuscript Preparation and Writing

11.1 Background

Manuscript writing is a skill that needs to be developed over time. It is important for submission and publication of your research work after completion of the research project. Conducting a sound research project and writing it scientifically are two different aspects, where many researchers find it difficult to put in their best interest. Unfortunately, the quality of research work is most importantly dependent on how well it is written and presented in the public domain. We can take 2 or 3 years to complete a research project with the highest level of dedication and precision, but the entire 3-year process does not necessarily be put through the manuscript. We have obvious limitations as there are prescribed formats, word limitations, and guidelines for writing different types of manuscripts. In this chapter, we will focus on important points while writing a case study, original article, and reviews. This is just a guideline while researchers are free to use their style of writing a manuscript. This chapter would help the researchers to prepare their research projects with a scientific representation and submission to journals for publication.

11.1.1 Writing a Case Study

A case study is a simple presentation of research findings for a single subject or a group of subjects through a "case series." Researchers need to understand that case studies in result have less evidence for the generalization of results to the masses and thus may lack applicability. In other words, research conducted on one case cannot be applied to all similar cases due to multifactorial differences. Moreover, as we learned, the scientific rigor in a case study would be limited and have research bias. However, unique cases or unreported cases of new diseases are useful for understanding the

A. Hazari, *Research Methodology for Allied Health Professionals*,
https://doi.org/10.1007/978-981-99-8925-6_11

basic nature of the problem and finding further research gaps. At the level of undergraduate in the allied health stream, case studies and case series may be opted for research projects. Although the case study would have all major sections of the resulting methodology, the emphasis would be given more on the subject progression on a day-to-day basis. Writing a case report starts with an introduction/background of the research while emphasizing the salient features of the case, previous literature, and the need to conduct the study. The introduction is usually followed by a "case description" where the detail of the subject is given clearly in the context of the research study. Under the methodology section, emphasis is given on the most important theme of the research as stated through the hypothesis. It could be a unique technique, unique finding, undiscovered complication, etc. The result section of the case study lacks inferential statistics, and mostly descriptive findings are presented. The result is followed by a brief discussion in the context of what and why the findings are important. Finally, a wider conclusion is drawn but not generalized. Case studies are generally reported within a limit of 1500 words. The international research experts have developed the CARE guidelines (for CAse REports) for increasing the accuracy and usefulness of case reports. Reachers could follow these guidleines available from Scientific Writing in Health and Medicine (SWIHM).

11.1.2 Writing an Original Article

Writing an original article is different from writing a case study in many ways. The original article is a representation of the entire research methodology used for the research project. It includes all components of research methodology in a scientific manner. The findings of the study can be used with confidence to generalize over the entire population. At the level of graduates/master programs in allied health streams, original research is preferred. While writing a manuscript, it is important to follow the widely accepted format for submission and publication as discussed below. The format may be commonly used for submission of any type of manuscript.

11.1.2.1 Preparation of Title Page

The title page of an original manuscript is separately asked by the journals during submission and includes the following:

- Title of Study: A complete title should be present at the top of the manuscript. Sometimes, a running title may be separately required by some journals.
- Author details: Here, the list of all authors should be given in order of affiliation. Contact details of the corresponding author are mandatorily required.
- Abstract: The abstract is a summary and reflection of the entire manuscript. The abstract can be "structured" or unstructured." The structured abstract has compo-

nents like background with aim, methodology, results, discussion, and conclusion briefly stated within a word limit of 200–500 words.
- Keywords: Four to five keywords are required which would be used to describe and search the manuscript
- Declaration of Interest: The author needs to declare any conflicts of interest.
- Declaration of Funding and Support: Any financial support for the study needs to be declared.
- Acknowledgment: Any nonfinancial support should be given in this section: for example, space and instrumentation.

11.1.2.2 Preparation of Cover Letter

In addition to the title page, the cover letter is requested by most journals. The cover letter should be addressed to the editor from the corresponding author. It should contain the title of the study and the journal name to which it is being submitted. The main body highlights the study's significance, which would match the scope of the journal.

11.1.2.3 Preparation of Main Text (Manuscript)

The main text of the original work is divided into major sections such as Introduction or Background, Methodology, Results, Discussion, Conclusion, and References. Ideally, a word limit of 2000–2500 is prescribed for most of the journal submissions. Therefore, it is very important for the researchers to precisely include all important points and to be concise in everything. The suggestions on how to write Introduction and Methodology have been given in previous chapters. Let us understand how to write the results, discussion, and conclusion in the manuscript.

Preparation of Results

Only the most important findings of the study need to be presented in this section. Tables and graphical presentations are often used to present the research findings with statistical data. Researchers need to understand that the data collection sheet does not need to be uploaded here. Also, the output tables from SPSS or any other software must NOT be uploaded in the result section. The results section should be self-explanatory, and statistical inferences should be given with p-value, confidence interval, effect size, etc. as per the objective of the study.

Preparation of Discussion

The discussion section of the manuscript is the most important part of writing. The section intends to discuss the findings of the study scientifically as per the objectives. The important findings of the study are reported here with justification on how and why those findings were obtained. Whether these findings are in line with previous research findings on similar topics, and if not, then what could be the possible scientific reason? The discussion should also explain the importance of the findings in context to its clinical implications (applicable for allied health professionals), industry applications, policy, planning, etc. It is important for researchers not to deviate from the main objectives of the study and to be consistent in elaborating their main findings with scientific justification. In the lack of any previous findings, researchers can use their professional knowledge to support their discussion points.

Preparation of Conclusion

The conclusion section of the manuscript is the final interpretation of the result findings. It should state whether the null hypothesis is rejected or accepted and how it could be applied to general findings. It is important for researchers not to conclude anything beyond their tested hypothesis and objectives.

Preparation of References

Acknowledging and giving respect to the original authors of the research are mandatory in manuscript writing. Any statement or idea drawn from other studies needs to be referenced in the Bibliography section after the conclusion and cited in the main text. There are various reference styles reported; we shall learn about them in the upcoming chapter.

11.1.3 Writing a Review

Writing a review study is different from original articles as here the entire process of research methodology is not executed. For example, there is no data collection procedure although data could be synthesized from previous literature. Review studies are most often conducted to establish an inference from previous literature. Review studies are compilations of important findings from previously published literature through "scoping reviews," "systematic reviews," and meta-analyses. Writing a manuscript for all review studies includes the same components from original research with an additional section for review of literature with details on systematic search strategy as explained in Chap. 7. The results section in the review studies focuses on the flow diagram and dataset for studies included in the review.

The discussion highlights important findings from each study with scientific justification, and the conclusion is made from all reviewed studies to justify the objective of conducting the review study. Reserchers in allied health stream often follow the PRISMA guidelines for reporting systematic reviews and metanalysis (http://prisma-statement.org/?AspxAutoDetectCookieSupport=1)

11.1.4 Summary

Scientific writing of a manuscript is different from general writing for blogs, non-scientific articles, advertisement articles, etc. Manuscript writing for research has defined sections and format. Researchers need to follow the instructions well for scientific writing and publication.

Chapter 12
Referencing: Use of Reference Manager

12.1 Background

Referencing in research is a critical aspect of academic writing. It involves citing the sources of information and ideas we have used in the research to give credit to the original authors and to enable readers to locate and verify the sources. Reference is the last component of research writing and should be done with accuracy. There are various referencing styles used in the research, and we will learn about them in this chapter. It is often difficult for the researchers to manage the references manually when the number is large. For such instances, researchers prefer to use reference managers, and we shall learn about them as well.

12.1.1 Need for Referencing

In research, referencing becomes essential from the ethical perspective where it is important to acknowledge the original intellectual work. Some of the important reasons for referencing are listed below:

12.1.1.1 Academic Integrity

Referencing enhances our commitment to academic honesty and integrity. It ascertains that the creators of the ideas, data, or concepts used in our research have been well credited and not shown as their self-credentials.

A. Hazari, *Research Methodology for Allied Health Professionals*,
https://doi.org/10.1007/978-981-99-8925-6_12

12.1.1.2 Building on Existing Knowledge

It weighs the contributions of other researchers and scholars in their field of expertise. Through referencing their work, we constantly upgrade our knowledge.

12.1.1.3 Verification and Replication

References allow readers to verify the information and arguments presented in the research. One can follow the citations to access the original sources and assess the accuracy and credibility of our work. This is essential for the peer-review process.

12.1.1.4 Avoiding Plagiarism

Plagiarism, which is the unauthorized use of someone else's work, is a serious ethical and academic offense. Proper referencing helps us avoid unintentional plagiarism.

12.1.1.5 Scientific Evidence and Support

While citing reputable and authoritative sources, we enhance our own credibility as a researcher. Readers are more likely to trust the work if we demonstrate that it is based on sound and well-established sources as the work would be supported through scientific evidence.

12.1.2 Referencing Styles

Multiple referencing styles are being used by the researchers, and each style has its own rules and formats for citing various types of sources in research papers and academic writing. We will learn about the most common referencing styles used by allied health professionals with examples. It is important to understand that each style has its own pattern for citation in the main text (short form) and the bibliography (full referencing). Let us learn a few commonly used referencing styles with the example given below.

12.1.2.1 Details of the Research: Example

Title: Kinetics and Kinematics of Diabetic Foot in Type 2 Diabetes Mellitus with and Without Peripheral Neuropathy: A Systematic Review and Meta-analysis

Authors: Animesh Hazari, Arun Maiya, Shivashankara K. N., Ioannis Agouris, Ashma Monteiro, Radhika Jadhav, Sampath Kumar, C. G. Shashi Kumar, and Shreemathi S. Mayya

Year of Publication: 2016

Journal Name: SpringerPlus

Volume: 5

Issue: 1

Page no.: 1–19

Let us learn to use this information for different referencing styles as discussed below. It is important to follow the sequence.

12.1.2.2 APA (American Psychological Association) Style

APA style is commonly used in the social sciences and includes both in-text citations and a references page.

In-text citation: In the manuscript text, only the name of the authors (surname) and year are given under the bracket as shown below. If there are three or more than three authors, then et al. is used followed by year of publication in brackets.

Worked examples for more than three authors: (Hazari et al., 2016)

Worked example for two authors: (Hazari & Maiya, 2016)

Worked example for single author: (Hazari, 2016)

APA Referencing in Bibliography:

- Surname followed by initial name and semicolon between each author
- – Full stop at the end of the author list
- – Followed by the year of publication in bracket and full stop
- – Followed by the title of the study and a full stop
- – Followed by the journal name and comma
- – Followed by volume and issue in bracket and comma
- – Followed by page no. starting–ending

Worked example: Hazari, A., Maiya, A. G., Shivashankara, K. N., Agouris, I., Monteiro, A., Jadhav, R., … & Mayya, S. S. (2016). Kinetics and kinematics of diabetic foot in type 2 diabetes mellitus with and without peripheral neuropathy: a systematic review and meta-analysis. Springerplus, 5(1), 1–19.

12.1.2.3 MLA (Modern Language Association) Style

MLA style is often used in humanities disciplines like literature and language studies.

In-text citation: In the manuscript text, only the name of the authors (surname) and year are given under the bracket as shown below. If there are three or more than three authors, then et al. is used followed by year of publication.

Worked examples for more than three authors: (Hazari et al., 2016)

Worked example for two authors: (Hazari and Maiya, 2016)
Worked example for single author: (Hazari, 2016)

MLA Referencing in Bibliography:

- Surname followed by initial name separated by the comma of the first author
  - Followed by et al. and full stop
  - Followed by "title of the study" and full stop
  - Followed by the journal name
  - Followed by volume and full stop followed by issue without bracket
  - Followed by the year of publication in bracket and
  - Followed by page no. starting–ending

Worked example: Hazari, Animesh, et al. "Kinetics and kinematics of diabetic foot in type 2 diabetes mellitus with and without peripheral neuropathy: a systematic review and meta-analysis." Springerplus 5.1 (2016): 1–19.

12.1.2.4 Chicago/Turabian Style

The Chicago style is used in history, while Turabian is a simplified version often used by students.

In-text citation: Same as above for MLA

Chicago Referencing in Bibliography:

- Surname followed by initial name and comma between each author
  - Full stop at the end of the author list
  - Followed by "title of the study" and full stop
  - Followed by the journal name
  - Followed by volume and full stop followed by issue without bracket
  - Followed by the year of publication in bracket and:
  - Followed by page no. starting–ending

Worked example: Hazari, Animesh, Arun G. Maiya, K. N. Shivashankara, Ioannis Agouris, Ashma Monteiro, Radhika Jadhav, Sampath Kumar, C. G. Shashi Kumar, and Shreemathi S. Mayya. "Kinetics and kinematics of diabetic foot in type 2 diabetes mellitus with and without peripheral neuropathy: a systematic review and meta-analysis." Springerplus 5, no. 1 (2016): 1–19.

12.1.2.5 Harvard Style

Harvard style is used in various disciplines and focuses on author year citations within the text and a reference list at the end.

In-text citation: Same as above for MLA

Harvard Referencing in Bibliography:

- Surname followed by initial name and semicolon between each author

- A semicolon (;) at the end of the author list
- Followed by the year of publication without bracket and full stop
- Followed by the title of the study and a full stop
- Followed by the journal name and comma
- Followed by volume and issue with bracket and comma
- Followed by pp. starting–ending

Worked example: Hazari, A., Maiya, A.G., Shivashankara, K.N., Agouris, I., Monteiro, A., Jadhav, R., Kumar, S., Shashi Kumar, C.G. and Mayya, S.S., 2016. Kinetics and kinematics of diabetic foot in type 2 diabetes mellitus with and without peripheral neuropathy: a systematic review and meta-analysis. Springerplus, 5(1), pp. 1–19.

12.1.2.6 Vancouver Style

The Vancouver style is commonly used in biomedical and scientific research.

In-text citation: Throughout, number is ordered and in brackets, e.g., [1]

Vancouver Referencing in Bibliography:

- Surname followed by initial name and comma between each author
- Full stop at the end of the author list
- Followed by the title of the study and a full stop
- Followed by the journal name and full stop
- Followed by the year of publication without a bracket
- Followed by the month and;
- Followed by volume and issue with bracket and:
- Followed by page no. starting–ending

Worked example: Hazari A, Maiya AG, Shivashankara KN, Agouris I, Monteiro A, Jadhav R, Kumar S, Shashi Kumar CG, Mayya SS. Kinetics and kinematics of diabetic foot in type 2 diabetes mellitus with and without peripheral neuropathy: a systematic review and meta-analysis. Springerplus. 2016 Dec;5(1):1–9.

12.1.3 Reference Managers

Also known as reference management software or citation managers, these are tools designed to help researchers organize, store, and format their references and citations. These tools are useful for maintaining a well-organized library of sources and for generating citations and bibliographies in various citation styles. The reference managers vary in terms of features, compatibility, and pricing. The choice of a reference manager often depends on your specific research needs, preferred citation style, and collaboration tools you require. It is essential to choose a reference manager that aligns with your research workflow and integrates well with your word processing software to streamline the citation and bibliography creation process. Some popular reference managers are listed below, and worked examples are shown for Mendeley, which is very commonly used by university students.

12.1.3.1 Zotero

It is a free, open-source reference manager that allows one to collect, organize, cite, and share research materials. It can automatically capture citation information from web pages, PDFs, and other sources. Zotero also integrates with word processing software like Microsoft Word and Google Docs for easy citation and bibliography creation.

12.1.3.2 EndNote

It is a widely used reference manager developed by Clarivate Analytics. It offers advanced features for organizing and managing references, including the ability to create custom reference types and organize references into groups. It is popular in scientific and medical research and requires a subscription for its use.

12.1.3.3 Mendeley

It is a free reference manager with social networking features. It allows you to organize PDFs, annotate documents, and collaborate with other researchers. It also integrates with Microsoft Word and LaTeX for citation and bibliography creation. We will learn the stepwise process to use Mendeley in the next section.

12.1.3.4 RefWorks

It is a web-based reference management tool often used by institutions and universities. It offers cloud-based storage, collaboration features, and various citation styles. It requires subscriptions and can support large research teams.

12.1.3.5 Citation Machine

While not a traditional reference manager, Citation Machine is an online tool that helps users generate citations and bibliographies in various citation styles. It is especially useful for quick citation generation when you do not need extensive reference management.

12.1.4 *Using Mendeley as Citation Manager*

As mentioned above, Mendeley is an easy and freely available citation manager used by many researchers. In this section, we shall learn how to cite and reference published articles on Mendeley. You would first need to register to Mendeley, following which you visit the Mendeley page as shown in Fig. 12.1 under the library section in the top right corner.

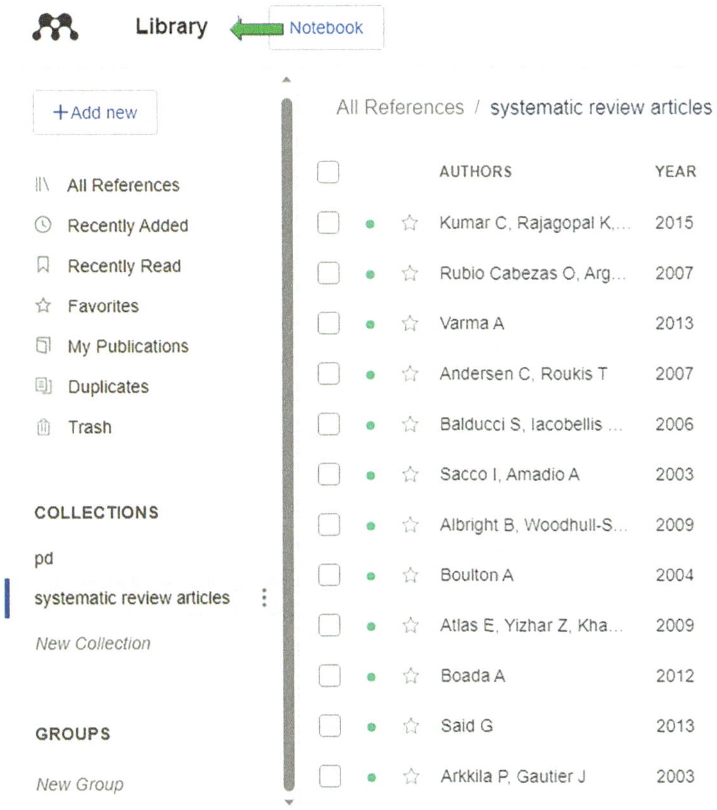

Fig. 12.1 Library section on the Mendeley home page

It would be advisable to create a desired research folder in the collection tab, and all articles could be put under it. In Fig. 12.2, we can see under the New Collection tab on the left sidebar that we have created a folder "Research Methods." Please note that the folder is blank, and now we will learn how to add the citation materials to this folder.

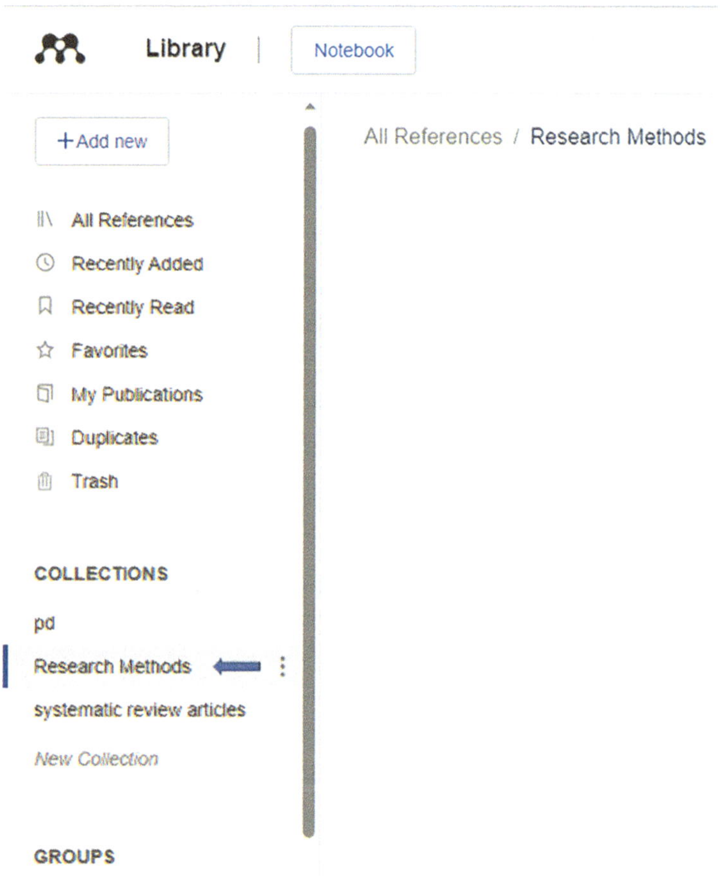

Fig. 12.2 New folder creation under the Collection tab.

To add any referencing material, click Add New on the top left corner of the page, and with any three options, viz. files from the computer, add an entry manually and import the library as shown in Fig. 12.3.

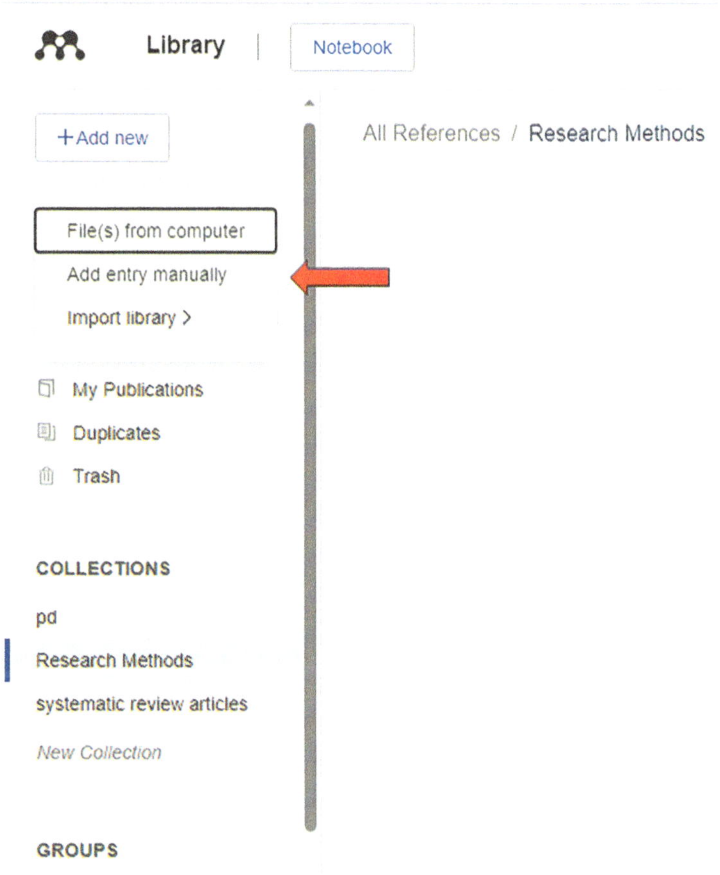

Fig. 12.3 Add options in the Mendeley library

Once all the referencing materials have been added, we will need to use the word plug-in option for citation and referencing in the Word file of the manuscript. To enable this, click on the "tools" tab on the top left corner of the page, and click "Install Mendeley Cite for Microsoft Word" as shown in Fig. 12.4.

Once you have downloaded the "Mendeley Cite" word plug-in, we can start our citation and referencing as discussed here. Open the Word document, click the reference tab, insert the citation where you wish to insert citation in the text, click Mendeley and it will take you to the Mendeley page, change the referencing style to the desired format, and click "cite" on Mendeley page as shown in Fig. 12.5. The citation would be automatically done in the desired format. For reference at the end of the manuscript, click "bibliography" in the reference tab of the Word document, and the references will appear automatically.

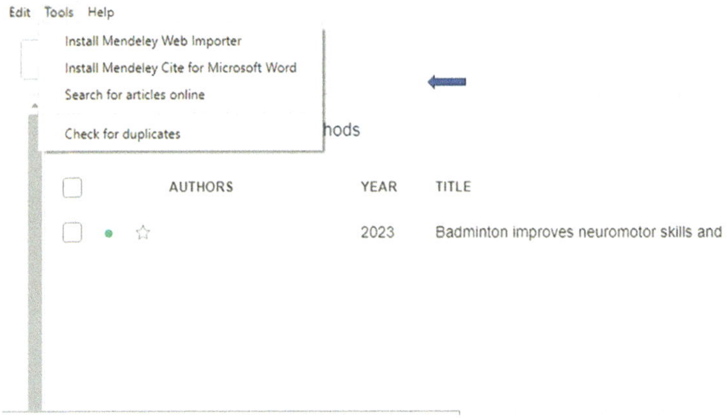

Fig. 12.4 Word plug-in system in the Mendeley

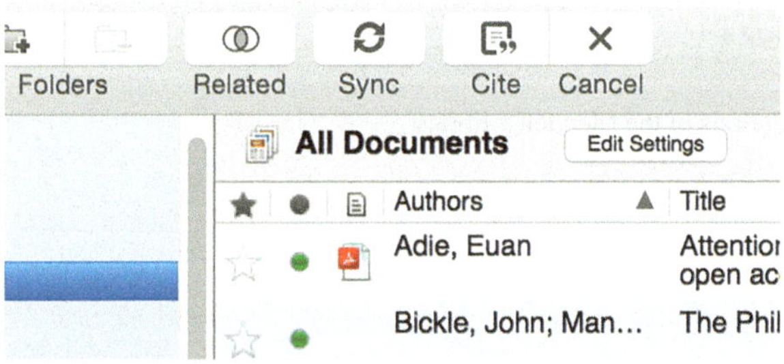

Fig. 12.5 Cite option in the Mendeley

12.1.5 Summary

Referencing is essential in research for self-credibility. In manuscripts, references are cited within the text and at the end of the manuscript section. Multiple reference managers could be used as per the availability and choice of the researcher. It is important to recheck the referencing list after using the referencing software for any error or discrepency.

Chapter 13
Selecting Journals for Publishing: Avoiding Rejection

13.1 Background

A well-written manuscript could be of no use when not available to readers publicly or unpublished. Journals and publication houses enable the work of researchers reach the designated community and identify their strengths as well as limitations. No one would have appreciated the work of Nikola Tesla or Einstein if their research papers were not published in reputable journals. There are multiple journals available, and publishing your hard work requires a comprehensive selection of the appropriate journal. Within the scope of the book for scientific research, we will learn how to select the correct journal for our research work publication.

13.1.1 Appropriate Journal for Your Work

The selection of the correct journal is an important part of the research publication process, and it depends upon the following salient points.

Type of research: It refers to whether we are looking to publish scientific or nonscientific research as the selection of journals would first depend on it. Also, types of research such as case studies, care reports, original articles, and reviews have specified journals for their publication and therefore should be submitted to respective journals only.

Abstract vs. full paper: Researchers can prefer to submit an abstract for publication before completion of the full manuscript; however, there are limited journals that offer abstract publication without full-text submission.

Target Audience: It is always important to understand the target audience before choosing the journal for publication. For example, if a work is related to educating the general masses, magazines, and newspapers would be appropriate whilst

A. Hazari, *Research Methodology for Allied Health Professionals*,
https://doi.org/10.1007/978-981-99-8925-6_13

avoiding advanced scientific concepts. However, if a research work relates to scientific findings targeted towards the research community, it should be published in scientific journals only as educated researchers would understand the scientific work.

Journal's scope of publication and thrust area: The selection of a journal essentially depends upon its scope and thrust area. A journal that aims to publish manuscripts in diabetic areas would not accept the submission of cancer research. Thus, when choosing a journal, it is always important to read the scope of the journal on its web page. If the scope matches our research work, it will be given due consideration for publication.

Journal Indexing and peer-review process: It is one of the most important points when choosing a journal for publication. Indexed journals are always preferred over non-indexed journals. The non-indexed journals are often predatory and published for monetary benefits without a peer-review process. They often do not follow the process of peer review for quick publication and therefore compromise with the quality of work. Indexed journals are rated high with higher visibility of the research work. The most reputed indexing sources are Scopus, Web of Science, PubMed, etc. Most research institutions make indexed publications mandatory for promotion and development. Therefore, due care should be taken while choosing indexed journals.

Journal Metrics and Article Processing Charges (APCs): It is always important for researchers to understand their level of research work and findings, which would ultimately determine the selection of a journal based on its metrics such as CiteScore, impact factor, Source Normalized Impact per Paper (SNIP), SCImago Journal Rank (SJR), h-index, and Quartile (Q1–Q4). The greater impact factor journals have high standards for publication and undergo rigorous screening and review. The Q1 journals hold higher citation metrics, and therefore the publication process is rigorous. Apart from that, many journals charge the publication fee as APC, and it depends upon the researcher to choose journals with APC or without APC. It should be noted that payment of APC does not guarantee publication, nor does it restrict the researcher from publishing their work in higher quartile journals without APC. Nowadays, open-access journals are available to release the research published immediately after publication to all readers without any restriction of subscriptions. The APC charges for open-access journals are paid by the researcher; however, there are provisions for requesting waiver or discount in APC, and researchers should explore the respective journal website for more information regarding this.

13.1.2 Avoiding Outright Rejection (Editorial Review)

When a manuscript is submitted, it undergoes the initial check for quality and standards for the journal from the editorial team. Following the initial check, the manuscript proceeds to the peer-review process. Therefore, it is important to understand the following common reasons for outright rejection at the level of editorial review.

- The title not matching the main text and objective.
- Conclusions do not support the hypothesis.
- Poor language comprehension.
- Frequent grammatical inaccuracy.
- Plagiarized work.
- Not meeting the formatting guidelines of the journal.
- Sources for conflict of interest.
- Ethical concerns.

13.1.3 Rejection at Peer Review

Manuscripts often suffer rejection at the peer-review level due to the following mistakes while preparing the manuscript sections.

Common Mistakes: Abstract
- Too much background or methods information
- Figures or images
- Abbreviations or acronyms
- Word limit exceeding

Common Mistakes: Introduction
- Too much or not enough information
- Unclear purpose and objective
- Confusing structure
- First-person anecdotes

Common Mistakes: Methodology
- Inappropriate study design and sampling error
- Wrong procedure of data collection
- Use of unstandardized methods and instrumentations
- Clear evidence of bias

Common Mistakes: Results
- Raw data without inference
- Data redundancy
- Wrong interpretation of data
- No figures or tables
- Methods/materials reported under result section

Common Mistakes: Discussion
- Combined with results
- Incorrectly discussing inconclusive results
- Ambiguous data sources
- Speculative assumptions
- Failure to justify the findings of the study scientifically

Common Mistakes: References

- Wrong format
- Wrong citations

13.1.4 Summary

It is important not only to conduct quality research work but also to write and select good journals for publication. The published research work provides higher visibility and reputation to the research work. Therefore, the correct selection of the journal is an essential step towards publication. Efforts should be made to avoid outright rejection in journals, and researchers must give due consideration to publishing in indexed, peer-reviewed journals.

Chapter 14
Critical Appraisal

14.1 Background

Critical appraisal is a systematic process used to evaluate the quality, validity, and relevance of research studies or articles. It is a fundamental step in evidence-based practice and helps researchers, healthcare professionals, and others assess the trustworthiness of research findings. Critical appraisal involves assessing various aspects of a study to determine its overall quality and whether its results can be applied to specific clinical or research questions. The purpose of critical appraisal is just to bring a critical review of the conducted and published work and not to purposely point out inaccuracy to establish one's own identity. It is similar to a critical review for any broadcast such as cinema, where experts evaluate all aspects to rate it. Similarly, a critical review of research is the evaluation of research through experts in that field. In this chapter, we will try to learn the components of research which are critically reviewed by the researchers and what the correct way to do so.

14.1.1 Review Components in Critical Appraisal

While conducting a critical appraisal, the following points are commonly assessed for their accuracy and applicability.

A. Hazari, *Research Methodology for Allied Health Professionals*,
https://doi.org/10.1007/978-981-99-8925-6_14

14.1.1.1 Study Design

Identifying the appropriate study design used in the research is essential. Therefore, the reviewer should be able to check the applicability of the study design used in the research work. Incorrect study design would not justify the findings and interpretation of the proposed hypothesis.

14.1.1.2 Sampling and Participants

Evaluating the methods used to select participants or subjects is important in research methodology. During critical appraisal, reviewers need to carefully determine whether the sample is representative of the target population and if there is any potential for selection bias.

14.1.1.3 Data Collection

For examining the data collection methods, including the use of valid and reliable measurement tools or instruments is a very important checklist for critical appraisal. It is also essential to assess the appropriateness of data collection procedures.

14.1.1.4 Data Analysis

In the process of critical appraisal, reviewing the statistical methods employed to analyze the data holds high significance. It is important to ensure that the statistical tests used are appropriate for the research question and that the results are accurately reported. The appropriate use of parametric and nonparametric tests enhances the accuracy of the research findings. In addition, assessing the potential for bias and confounding variables that could affect the study results is very important. It would be important to look for efforts made by the researchers to minimize these issues to report the results.

14.1.1.5 Presentation of Results and Findings

For examining the presentation of results, including the use of tables, figures, and text is an essential aspect of the critical appraisal process. Reviewers must check whether the results are clearly reported and whether they answer the research question appropriately.

14.1.1.6 Conclusion

Evaluating the authors' interpretation of the results during the critical appraisal is the most important point. Researchers often come to conclusions that may be over-optimistic, not supported by their findings, and beyond the scope of the study. Therefore, it is important to determine whether the conclusions are supported by the evidence presented in the study.

14.1.1.7 Ethical Considerations

Ensure that the study is adhered to ethical principles and guidelines by including informed consent, protection of human subjects, and disclosure of conflicts of interest.

14.1.1.8 Study Quality Checklist

Researchers often rate the quality of studies using checklists. In the allied health profession, the Downs and Black checklist could be used with higher applicability and effectiveness (Downs and Black 1998). There are other checklists also available which could be used to assess the quality of the studies.

14.1.2 Reporting Guidelines and Critical Appraisal Tools

There are various reporting guidelines and critical appraisal tool checklists available for specific study designs (e.g., CONSORT for RCTs, STROBE for observational studies). These tools can provide a structured approach to evaluating a study. Researchers can follow the JBI and EQUATOR checklists for critical appraisal of various study designs. It is freely available for research purposes and is most widely used by researchers in allied health professions. The JBI checklist for RCTs, systematic reviews, and qualitative, prevalence, and cross-sectional studies have been given in Appendixes 14.1–14.5 for your reference.

14.1.3 Summary

Critical appraisal is an essential skill for researchers, healthcare professionals, and anyone using research evidence to inform decisions. It helps ensure that the best available evidence is used to support decision-making and promotes the use of high-quality research in various fields.

Appendixes

Appendix 14.1: JBI Critical Appraisal Checklist for Randomized Controlled Trials (Tufanaru et al. 2020)

Reviewer ______________________________________

Date ______________________________

Author _______________________________________ Year _________

Record Number _________

	Yes	No	Unclear	NA
1. Was true randomization used for assignment of participants to treatment groups?	☐	☐	☐	☐
2. Was allocation to treatment groups concealed?	☐	☐	☐	☐
3. Were treatment groups similar at the baseline?	☐	☐	☐	☐
4. Were participants blind to treatment assignment?	☐	☐	☐	☐
5. Were those delivering treatment blind to treatment assignment?	☐	☐	☐	☐
6. Were outcome assessors blind to treatment assignment?	☐	☐	☐	☐
7. Were treatment groups treated identically other than the intervention of interest?	☐	☐	☐	☐
8. Was follow-up complete, and if not, were differences between groups in terms of their follow-up adequately described and analyzed?	☐	☐	☐	☐
9. Were participants analyzed in the groups to which they were randomized?	☐	☐	☐	☐
10. Were outcomes measured in the same way for treatment groups?	☐	☐	☐	☐
11. Were outcomes measured in a reliable way?	☐	☐	☐	☐
12. Was appropriate statistical analysis used?	☐	☐	☐	☐
13. Was the trial design appropriate, and have any deviations from the standard RCT design (individual randomization, parallel groups) been accounted for in the conduct and analysis of the trial?	☐	☐	☐	☐

Overall appraisal: Include ☐ Exclude ☐ Seek further info ☐

Comments (Including reason for exclusion)

Appendix 14.2: JBI Critical Appraisal Checklist for Systematic Reviews and Research Syntheses (Aromataris et al. 2015)

Reviewer ______________________________________

Date ______________________________

Author _______________________________________ Year _________

Record Number _________

	Yes	No	Unclear	Not applicable
14. Is the review question clearly and explicitly stated?	☐	☐	☐	☐
15. Were the inclusion criteria appropriate for the review question?	☐	☐	☐	☐
16. Was the search strategy appropriate?	☐	☐	☐	☐
17. Were the sources and resources used to search for studies adequate?	☐	☐	☐	☐
18. Were the criteria for appraising studies appropriate?	☐	☐	☐	☐
19. Was critical appraisal conducted by two or more reviewers independently?	☐	☐	☐	☐
20. Were there methods to minimize errors in data extraction?	☐	☐	☐	☐
21. Were the methods used to combine studies appropriate?	☐	☐	☐	☐
22. Was the likelihood of publication bias assessed?	☐	☐	☐	☐
23. Were recommendations for policy and/or practice supported by the reported data?	☐	☐	☐	☐
24. Were the specific directives for new research appropriate?	☐	☐	☐	☐

Overall appraisal: Include ☐ Exclude ☐ Seek further info ☐

Comments (Including reason for exclusion)

____

____

____

Appendix 14.3: JBI Critical Appraisal Checklist for Qualitative Research (Lockwood et al. 2015)

Reviewer ____________________________________

Date _____________________________

Author _____________________________________ Year ________

Record Number ________

	Yes	No	Unclear	Not applicable
25. Is there congruity between the stated philosophical perspective and the research methodology?	☐	☐	☐	☐
26. Is there congruity between the research methodology and the research question or objectives?	☐	☐	☐	☐
27. Is there congruity between the research methodology and the methods used to collect data?	☐	☐	☐	☐
28. Is there congruity between the research methodology and the representation and analysis of data?	☐	☐	☐	☐

	Yes	No	Unclear	Not applicable
29. Is there congruity between the research methodology and the interpretation of results?	☐	☐	☐	☐
30. Is there a statement locating the researcher culturally or theoretically?	☐	☐	☐	☐
31. Is the influence of the researcher on the research, and vice versa, addressed?	☐	☐	☐	☐
32. Are participants, and their voices, adequately represented?	☐	☐	☐	☐
33. Is the research ethical according to current criteria or, for recent studies, is there evidence of ethical approval by an appropriate body?	☐	☐	☐	☐
34. Do the conclusions drawn in the research report flow from the analysis, or interpretation, of the data?	☐	☐	☐	☐

Overall appraisal: Include ☐ Exclude ☐ Seek further info ☐

Comments (Including reason for exclusion)

____

____

____

Appendix 14.4: JBI Critical Appraisal Checklist for Studies Reporting Prevalence Data (Munn et al. 2015)

Reviewer ______________________

Date ______________________

Author ______________________ Year ________

Record Number ________

	Yes	No	Unclear	Not applicable
35. Was the sample frame appropriate to address the target population?	☐	☐	☐	☐
36. Were study participants sampled in an appropriate way?	☐	☐	☐	☐
37. Was the sample size adequate?	☐	☐	☐	☐
38. Were the study subjects and the setting described in detail?	☐	☐	☐	☐
39. Was the data analysis conducted with sufficient coverage of the identified sample?	☐	☐	☐	☐
40. Were valid methods used for the identification of the condition?	☐	☐	☐	☐
41. Was the condition measured in a standard, reliable way for all participants?	☐	☐	☐	☐
42. Was there appropriate statistical analysis?	☐	☐	☐	☐

	Yes	No	Unclear	Not applicable
43. Was the response rate adequate, and if not, was the low response rate managed appropriately?	☐	☐	☐	☐

Overall appraisal: Include ☐ Exclude ☐ Se
ek further info ☐
Comments (Including reason for exclusion)

____
____
____

Appendix 14.5: JBI Critical Appraisal Checklist for Analytical Cross-Sectional Studies (Moola et al. 2020)

Reviewer ______________________________
Date ________________________
Author ______________________________ Year _______
Record Number _______

	Yes	No	Unclear	Not applicable
1. Were the criteria for inclusion in the sample clearly defined?	☐	☐	☐	☐
2. Were the study subjects and the setting described in detail?	☐	☐	☐	☐
3. Was the exposure measured in a valid and reliable way?	☐	☐	☐	☐
4. Were objective, standard criteria used for measurement of the condition?	☐	☐	☐	☐
5. Were confounding factors identified?	☐	☐	☐	☐
6. Were strategies to deal with confounding factors stated?	☐	☐	☐	☐
7. Were the outcomes measured in a valid and reliable way?	☐	☐	☐	☐
8. Was appropriate statistical analysis used?	☐	☐	☐	☐

Overall appraisal: Include ☐ Exclude ☐ Se
ek further info ☐
Comments (Including reason for exclusion)

____
____
____
____
____

References

Aromataris E, Fernandez R, Godfrey C, Holly C, Kahlil H, Tungpunkom P. Summarizing systematic reviews: methodological development, conduct and reporting of an Umbrella review approach. Int J Evid Based Healthc. 2015;13(3):132-40.

Downs, S. H., & Black, N. (1998). The feasibility of creating a checklist for the assessment of the methodological quality both of randomised and non-randomised studies of health care interventions. Journal of Epidemiology and Community Health, 52(6), 377–384. https://doi.org/10.1136/jech.52.6.377

Lockwood C, Munn Z, Porritt K. Qualitative research synthesis: methodological guidance for systematic reviewers utilizing meta-aggregation. Int J Evid Based Healthc. 2015;13(3):179–187.

Moola S, Munn Z, Tufanaru C, Aromataris E, Sears K, Sfetcu R, Currie M, Qureshi R, Mattis P, Lisy K, Mu P-F. Chapter 7: Systematic reviews of etiology and risk. In: Aromataris E, Munn Z (Editors). JBI Manual for Evidence Synthesis. JBI, 2020.

Munn Z, Moola S, Lisy K, Riitano D, Tufanaru C. Methodological guidance for systematic reviews of observational epidemiological studies reporting prevalence and incidence data. Int J Evid Based Healthc. 2015;13(3):147–153.

Tufanaru C, Munn Z, Aromataris E, Campbell J, Hopp L. Chapter 3: Systematic reviews of effectiveness. In: Aromataris E, Munn Z (Editors). JBI Manual for Evidence Synthesis. JBI, 2020.

Chapter 15
Ethics in Research Methodology

15.1 Background

Ethical practices are important to ensure the integrity of values in research. There are multiple instances where the ethical principles come into play for researchers. An ethical approach may be harder, but the outcome is fruitful. All research needs to seek approval from the ethical board, thereby safeguarding the welfare of all. Ethics in research refers to the moral principles and guidelines that researchers must adhere to when conducting studies involving human subjects, animals, or other sensitive areas of inquiry. Ethics in research has a broader meaning where not only the researchers but also the participants must regulate the laws of ethical practice. In this chapter, we will learn the common instances of unethical practices or breaches of ethical practices.

15.1.1 Breach of Information

This is one of the most common breaches in ethical practice by the researcher in health sciences. As per the Declaration of Helsinki, there is a law to protect the well-being of human subjects involved in biomedical research; however, at times, researchers may hide sensitive information from the ethical committee for ease in the approval process. Besides, the researcher may not provide adequate information to the subjects about the research study for certain benefits, and this would be considered as an unethical practice. The ethical considerations are often neglected with not providing either the informed consent or the participant information sheet or both to the subjects. Researchers need to understand the difference between an informed consent form and a participant information sheet. The informed consent is a brief document stating the title and participant's willingness to participate under

A. Hazari, *Research Methodology for Allied Health Professionals*,
https://doi.org/10.1007/978-981-99-8925-6_15

the supervision of the researcher, undersigned, whereas the participant information sheet is a detailed copy of the research detail and its various aspects. A common performance for information sheet and participant information sheet has been worked out as examples in Appendixes 15.1 and 15.2. There can be slight differences in the template from institution to institution, but the main sections remain the same.

15.1.2 Breach in Sample Recruitment

There can be an ethical breach in the data collection process from both the researcher and participant end. Researchers often drift towards proving their research hypothesis and purposely select participants who would best fit into it to yield desired results. At times, participants also want themselves to be selected for the research for certain benefits, which may not fall into the standards of research methodology and would be considered as an unethical practice in research.

15.1.3 Breach in Data Collection Procedure

For interventional studies, data collection procedures become difficult, and researchers may unintentionally breach ethics in research. For example, where the control group is present and depriving them of the particular treatment option would be unethical. Researchers should ensure that the selection of participants is fair and equitable. This enables avoiding discrimination and ensuring that vulnerable populations are not exploited or disproportionately burdened by research.

15.1.4 Breach of Beneficence

To adhere to the ethics in research, investigators should aim to maximize benefits and minimize harm to participants. They must carefully assess the potential risks and benefits of the research and take steps to ensure that the benefits outweigh the risks or else it would be considered as an unethical practice.

15.1.5 Breach of Privacy and Confidentiality

Researchers need to respect the privacy of participants and maintain the confidentiality of their data. This includes protecting sensitive information and ensuring that participant's identities are not disclosed without their consent. Use of pictures, statements, videos, etc. of the patient for manuscript publication is also an unethical practice if done without permission from the concerned.

15.1.6 Breach of Autonomy

Researchers must respect the autonomy and self-determination of participants. This allows participants to make their own decisions about participation and ensure that they are not coerced or manipulated in any way.

15.1.7 Breach of Integrity and Honesty

Researchers should conduct their work with honesty and integrity, accurately reporting their findings and avoiding fabrication, falsification, or plagiarism. Plagiarism in research is one of the most serious ethical considerations. It refers to stealing the original work without giving proper credit to the owners of the intellectual property. Researchers often do extensive paraphrasing of published work, which would still be considered as an unethical practice. Therefore, intentionally, we must avoid replicating others' work and try to maintain originality.

15.1.8 Role of Institutional Review Board (IRB)

All research institutions have IRBs that review research proposals to ensure that they meet ethical standards. Researchers first present their proposal to the IRB and must obtain IRB approval before conducting studies involving human subjects. Few institutions have ethical committees separately to look only at the ethical aspects of the research.

15.1.9 Summary

Ethical considerations in research are not static and may evolve. Researchers should stay informed about current ethical guidelines and best practices in their respective fields and disciplines. Violating ethical principles in research can have serious consequences, including damage to the reputation of the researcher and potential legal and ethical repercussions. Therefore, ethical conduct is paramount in all stages of the research methodology.

Appendixes

Appendix 15.1: Model for Informed Consent Form

Informed Consent Form (English)

Project title: Foot Kinematics and Kinetics in Type 2 Diabetes Mellitus with and Without Peripheral Neuropathy

Research Subject Id:

Age of the Research Subject (to be taken from parents if minor):

I have read the Participant Information Sheet and its contents were explained. I had the opportunity to ask questions and received satisfactory answers.

I understand that my participation in the study is voluntary and that I have the right to withdraw at any time without giving any reason, without my medical care or legal rights being affected.

I agree to take part in the above study. I confirm that I have received a copy of the Participant Information Sheet along with this signed and dated informed consent form.

__________________________ _________

Signature of the research subject Date

__________________________ _________

Name of the research subject Date

__________________________ _________

Signature and the name of the witness Date

__________________________ _________

Signature of the person explaining the consent Date

Appendix 15.2: Model for Participant Information Sheet

Model Participant Information Sheet (English)

Protocol title: Foot Kinematics and Kinetics in Type 2 Diabetes Mellitus with and Without Peripheral Neuropathy

Principal Investigator: Animesh Hazari

Designation: PhD Scholar

Hospital: KH, Department of Physiotherapy

Contact number: xxx

Please read this form carefully. If you do not understand the language or any information in this document, please discuss with study doctor. If you decide to volunteer to take part in this study, you must sign at the end of this form.

1. Introduction to the research study:

You are being asked to take part in this study because you have been diagnosed with type 2 diabetes mellitus, and this study involves the use of a biomechanical assessment tool for detecting complications of foot in type 2 diabetes mellitus participants. This instrument is approved by concerned authority and has no harmful effects.

2. Purpose of the study:

   To determine and identify various risk factors that lead to alteration in foot biomechanics and resultant foot complication in type 2 diabetes mellitus

3. Who can take part:

   Age group of 35–70 years

   Gender: male and female both

   Type 2 diabetes mellitus with and without neuropathy

4. Information about the study:

   A total of 600 subject participants will participate in the study. A general screening procedure for diabetic foot complications shall be done by the physical therapist. After this, data collection will be done. Proper safety precautions for diabetes control will be taken.

5. What will happen during the study (plan of action during the study)

   The participant will be called only once to KH, and demographic information will be taken, whereas participant will be thoroughly explained about the rules and regulations of the study. The physical examination will include general screening procedure like dermatologic, neurological, musculoskeletal, and vascular components.

6. Your role/responsibility in the study (role of the participant during the study):

   Please provide accurate information, and take part in the study with enthusiasm. Any discomfort during the study needs to be mentioned.

7. What are the risks?

   There is no potential risk associated with the study. However, necessary steps like juice and sweet will be made available for hypoglycemic control.

8. What are the potential benefits of participating in the study:

   You may or may not get benefit from participating in this study. If you take part in this study, you may help other patients with type 2 diabetes by contributing to the knowledge about risk factors and complications of foot.

9. Cost of participating in the study:

   Tests and procedures required for the study are provided at no cost to you.

10. Compensation for injury:

    If a medical problem arises during this research study as a direct result of the study treatment, the study doctor will be responsible for making sure that proper medical care is provided to you.

11. Confidentiality of information:

    Information from the study including your name, address, medical records, results of tests, and study results will be reviewed only by authorized personnel from the sponsor or their representative, ethics committee, or regulatory bodies. Information and results from this study may be presented at meetings or published in journals without including your name and personal identification.

12. New information about the study:

    Any new information available during the study will be informed to you if it has relevance to your decision regarding continuing in the study.

13. Voluntary participation:

    Entering a research study is voluntary. If you volunteer for a research study, you have the right to stop at any time and you need not give any reason for the same. Your decision not to participate in the study will not affect your future treatment. Sponsor or the investigator may stop the research or your participation in it at any time for some or other reason without your permission.

14. Whom to contact in case of any questions:

    If you have any questions about this form or any study-related issue, you may contact the following person (he/she should not be involved in the research directly):

    Name:

    Address:

    Telephone No.:

15. Signature of the participant

Date:

The manufacturer's authorised representative in the EU is Springer Nature Customer Service Centre GmbH, Europaplatz 3, 69115 Heidelberg, Germany. If you have any concerns regarding our products, please contact ProductSafety@springernature.com

Printed and bound by CPI Group (UK) Ltd, Croydon, CR0 4YY
01/10/2026
02225916-0010